SOUL TO SOUL

xo
mom

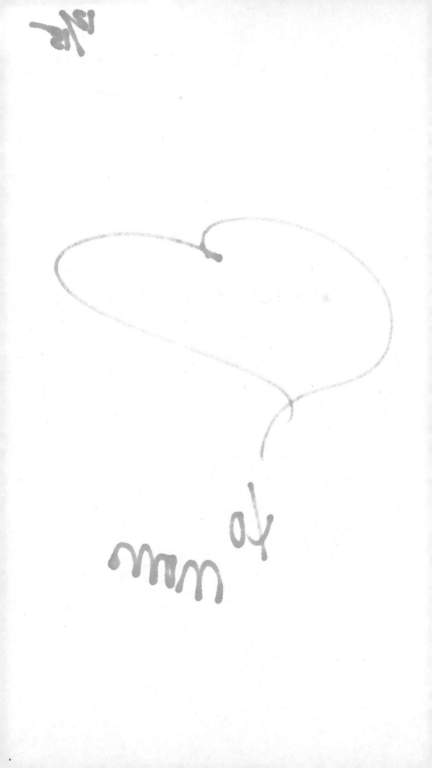

SOUL TO SOUL

POEMS, PRAYERS AND STORIES TO END A YOGA CLASS

COMPILED AND EDITED BY
JOHN MUNDAHL

RED ELIXIR/MONKFISH BOOK PUBLISHING COMPANY
RHINEBECK, NEW YORK

Soul To Soul: Poems, Prayers and Stories to End a Yoga Class ©
2010, 2015 compiled and edited by John Mundahl

Printed in the United States of America

Library of Congress Control Number: 2010901245

Paperback ISBN: 978-1-939681-42-3
eBook ISBN: 978-1-939681-46-1

Red Elixir—A Body, Mind, Spirit Imprint of Monkfish
22 East Market Street, Suite 304
Rhinebeck, New York 12572
www.monkfishpublishing.com
USA 845-876-4861

FOREWORD
By Yogi Amrit Desai

THE PURPOSE OF YOGA is manifold, but its ultimate aim is integration—integration of body, mind, heart and soul. It is only through harmony and oneness that we can attain even a glimpse of the cosmic divine soul that we are. With continued practice and dedication, integration deepens and direct experiences of our own divinity become more profound.

It is my privilege and pleasure to endorse the work of John Mundahl, both in his own search for unity and in his untiring efforts at providing that experience to others through his books. The closing of a yoga class is a sacred moment. It can dissolve in an instant, if the mind darts to the busy-ness of the day ahead, the snarled traffic or the many inconveniences of modern life. If captured and held close in our heart, that moment in time can sustain us through these very annoyances that disturb our peace and disrupt our ability to stay connected to the Source. It is my hope that this compilation of inspired readings will enhance your yoga practice, deepen the integration of your being and bring you closer to the Soul.

INTRODUCTION

A SPECIAL PART of each yoga class is the relaxation period on the end, when everyone lies flat on the floor, covers themselves, and is led into an experience of deep rest. It is called *savasana* in yoga and it is an important part of any yoga class.

Why is this so? Because the yoga postures practiced during class are designed to release tension and blocks in the body and mind of the practitioner so that *prana*, the life force, is free to heal. This healing occurs most powerfully at the end of each class during *savasana*.

The selections in this book can be read during *savasana*, or at the end of *savasana*, and will help in the healing process. Not all of the selections are serious, as humor and light heartedness should surely be a part of our spiritual journey.

I've been a yoga teacher and practitioner for 32 years and have always wanted just one book that I could bring to class with enough meaningful readings for everyone. Hopefully this will be such a book. The book was inspired, as always, by my two yoga teachers and spiritual guides, Swami Kripalu, a master of Shaktipat Kundalini Yoga, and his spiritual son, Yogi Amrit Desai, and I am once again endebted to them for their vast influence on my life. I was fortunate to be a resident at the original Kripalu Yoga Ashram from 1977-1981, the four years of Swami Kripalu's remarkable stay in the United States and it altered my life.

I never intended to write any selections for this book, but I discovered that publishing houses want money to quote material from the books they control (light bulb!). So after I had put together the original anthology, I found that I couldn't afford it, and I began deleting selections and writing my own to keep to my goal of 150 selections.

Hopefully the book will be a blessing to you.

"Don't think that only saints can give blessings," Swami Kripalu told us when he was with us in the United States. "Anyone can give a blessing. A blessing comes from the heart and thus from God."

So this book comes from my heart to yours. May your quest for peace, health and happiness be fulfilled.

Hari Om, Shanti, Shanti, Shanti.

John Mundahl, 2010
Edina, Minnesota

DEDICATION

*In loving memory of Margaret Irene Mundahl,
1917-1967, my mother and first yoga teacher.*

May her soul be filled with joy.

TABLE OF CONTENTS

SOUL TO SOUL

Poems, Prayers and Stories
to End a Yoga Class

INVOCATION

May He who is Father in Heaven to the Christians,
Holy One to the Jews,
Allah to the Muslims,
Buddha to the Buddhists,
Tao to the Chinese,
Ahura Mazda to the Zoroastrians,
Great Spirit to the Native Peoples,
And Brahma to the Hindus,
Lead us from the unreal to the Real,
From darkness to light,
From disease and death to immortality.
May the All-Loving Being manifest Himself to us,
And grant us abiding understanding
And all-consuming divine love.
Hari Om, Shanti. Shanti. Shanti.
Peace. Peace. Peace be unto all.

Swami Akhilananda, 1894-1962
Bangladesh

1

The Sun Never Says *by Hafiz*

Even
After
All this time
The sun never says to the earth,

"You owe
Me."

Look
What happens
With a love like that,
It lights the
Whole
Sky.

"We are born for love…It is the principle of existence and its only end." Disraeli

True Love Is For Fools *by Swami Kripalu*

Usually what we call love isn't love.
True love never ends.
Once the flame of true love is lit,
It can never be put out.
It doesn't start and stop,
Sometimes on, sometimes off.
It's always giving and serving, no matter what.
This is its nature.

One who can't tolerate pain
Can't travel on the path of true love.
True love is for fools.
They are fools to the desires of the world,
So worldly people call them fools.
But they aren't fools, really.

They're simply full of love.

Close your eyes
And draw all your senses inward
And enter the depth of your heart
And ask yourself:
Have I ever experienced this kind of love from anybody?
It's so rare.

"Love is always open arms. If you close your arms about love, you will find that you are left holding only yourself." Leo Buscaglia

The Man With The Funny Yoga Mat

by John Mundahl

Once a man came to my yoga class.
The first day he walked up to me and said,
 "I need exercise. Will I get that here?"
 "Yes," I said. "Yoga is exercise."
He was blunt and direct and walked away.
I watched him spread out his yoga mat,
But I could see that the mat wouldn't lie flat.
The edges were curled up.

The next week he came up to me and said,
 "I'm sleeping better. But I don't want to give up ice
 cream."
 "That's fine," I said.
He walked away and
I watched him spread out his yoga mat.
The edges were still curled up,
But I could see that his mat was trying to lie flat.

The next week he came but he was quiet.
He only spoke to me after class.
 "What is this anyway?"
 "What is what?" I asked.
 "Yoga."
 "It's what you want it to be," I said.
He was puzzled, but curious,
And I watched him walk out the door,
Yoga mat under his arm.

The next week he came and said,
 "I'm losing some of this!"

He shook his belly a bit
And laughed for the first time.
    "That's good," I said.
He spread out his yoga mat
And I could see that the edges were starting to lie flat.

On the last day of class
He came up to me with a soft face.
    "There was a beautiful sunset last night. Did you see it?"
    "Yes," I said. "I saw it."
Then he walked away,
To a quiet corner of the classroom
And spread out his yoga mat
And the edges were flat
And his yoga mat lie flat.

"Yoga is our natural state. We just have to rediscover it. We had it as children. We lost it as we grew up and took on the world."
Anonymous

4

The Paradox Of Our Age *by the Dalai Lama*

We have bigger houses but smaller families;
More conveniences, but less time.
We have more degrees, but less sense;
More knowledge, but less judgment
More experts, but more problems;
More medicines, but less healthiness;
We've been all the way to the moon and back,
But have trouble crossing the street to meet the new
neighbor.
We built more computers to hold more
Information to produce more copies than ever,
But have less communication;
We have become long on quantity,
But short on quality.
These are times of fast food
But slow digestion;
Tall man but short character;
Steep profits but shallow relationships.
It's a time when there is much in the window
But nothing in the room.

"It's not enough to be busy, so are the ants. The question is: What are we busy about?" Henry David Thoreau

5

Wouldn't It Be Funny *by Yogi Amrit Desai*

Wouldn't it be funny if trees were sad in the fall
Because the leaves were gone?

Wouldn't it be funny if lakes were sad in the winter
Because they were covered with ice?

Wouldn't it be funny if flowers were sad in the spring
Because they had to close up at night?

Wouldn't it be funny if rain was sad in the summer
Because rainbows had to end?

Nothing works that way in nature.
What is…simply is.

No judgment, just acceptance.
The hillside is peaceful whether covered with flowers or
snow.

"My secret?" J. Krishnamurte said. "I don't mind what happens."

Beauty Arises In The Stillness Of Your Presence
by Eckhart Tolle

Beyond the beauty of the external forms there is more
here:
Something that can't be named, something ineffable,
Some deep, inner, holy essence.

Whenever and wherever there is beauty,
This inner essence shines through somehow.
It only reveals itself to you when you are present.
Mind, which lives in the past or future,
Can neither recognize nor create beauty.

Could it be that this nameless essence and your presence
Are one and the same thing?
Would it be there without your presence?
Go deeply into it.
Find out for yourself.

"Come out of the circle of time and into the circle of love." Rumi

Yoga, On The Other Hand *by Dr. David Frawley*

O UR VERY WAY of life breeds unhappiness. We have an active and turbulent culture in which there is little peace or contentment. We have disturbed the organic roots of life, which are good food, water, air and a happy family life. We live in an artificial world dominated by an urban landscape and mass media, in which there is little to nourish the soul.

We ever desire new things and are seldom content with what we have. We run from one stimulation to another, rarely observing the process of our lives that is really leading nowhere.

Our lives are patterns of accumulation in which we are never still or at rest. Our medicine is more of a quick fix to keep us going in our wrong lifestyles and seldom addresses the behavioral root of our problems. We take a quick pill hoping that our problem will go away, not recognizing that it may only be a symptom of a life out of balance, like a warning light that we had better heed.

Yoga, on the other hand, teaches harmony with Nature, simplicity and contentment as keys to well being. It shows us how to live in a state of balance in which fulfillment is a matter of being, not becoming. It connects us with the wellsprings of creativity and happiness within our own consciousness, so that we can permanently overcome our psychological problems.

Yoga provides a real solution to our health problems, which is to return to oneness with both the universe and the Divine within. This requires changing how we live, think and perceive.

"Before you practice yoga, the theory is useless. After you practice yoga, the theory is obvious." David Williams

8

A Practice For Touching Peace *by Thich Nhat Hanh*

CONSCIOUS BREATHING is the most basic Buddhist practice for touching peace. I would like to offer you this short exercise:

> *Breathing in, I calm my body.*
> *Breathing out, I smile.*
> *Dwelling in the present moment,*
> *I know this is a wonderful moment.*

"Breathing in, I calm my body." This is like drinking a glass of cool water. You feel the freshness permeate your body. "Breathing out, I smile." One smile can relax hundreds of muscles in your face and make you master of yourself. Whenever you see a picture of the Buddha, He is always smiling. "Dwelling in the present moment." We recite this line as we breathe in again and we don't think of anything else. We know exactly where we are. "I know this is a wonderful moment." We recite this as we breathe out again.

To be truly here now and to enjoy the present moment is our most important task.

"When you inhale, you are taking the strength from God. When you exhale, it represents the service you are giving to the world."
B.K.S. Iyengar

My Soul Mate, Where Are You? *by John Mundahl*

Today I stopped to look with shy eyes
Around the corner to see if you were there,
Hoping at last to find you. But I was left alone again
To wonder if we will ever meet.

I looked afar toward flowered hills, as well,
And stretched out my hand in love toward you,
Hoping at last to feel your touch. But I was left alone
again
To wonder if we will ever meet.

I sat next to flowing mountain stream
And listened to soothing sound of water over rocks,
Hoping at last to hear your voice. But I was left alone
again
To wonder if we will ever meet.

Then a bird, fresh with spring, sang to me,
And you, my love, burst with tender eyes from deep
within my heart.
You wrapped me in your arms and held me and wiped
my tears
And I knew I would never be alone again.

*"When ignorance is destroyed, the Self is liberated from its
identification with the world. This liberation is Enlightenment."
The Yoga Sutras of Patanjali.*

10

You Cannot Receive Love When Your Heart Is Clenched *by Dr. Henry Emmons*

J OY IS NOT the absence of suffering, nor the opposite of sadness. Joy is simply the natural outcome of *knowing* and *feeling* the connection that your soul longs for. It isn't an object or an achievement. It's more like a gentle breeze that simply comes, on its own, when it's allowed to do so. But if joy is really natural, why doesn't it come to us more often and more easily?

Usually joy is not present because we haven't allowed it to be. We block it chemically, with unbalanced bio-chemicals in our brain, with poor nutrition that depletes our bodies, or sleep patterns that disrupt our relationship to nature and our own cycles.

We block it with our thoughts, when we strive to control the uncontrollable, to grasp after happiness, to push away love and connection, to blind ourselves to internal and external reality.

We block it with our hearts, too, when we close down in fear or resentment or confusion. You cannot receive an object when your hand is clenched. You cannot receive food when your jaws are clenched. You cannot receive joy when your mind is clenched. And you cannot receive love when your heart is clenched.

"When I stopped comparing myself to others in class, I started to like yoga. I realized it wasn't about them and me; it was about what was happening inside my body. Was I comfortable with my body or not? Could I accept myself or not? Really, it's a journey inward, not outward." Anonymous

11

If The Buddha Dated *by Charlotte Kasl*

W HAT WOULD IT MEAN to bring a Buddha consciousness to dating? Instead of feeling a sense of urgency, we would be fascinated by the process of meeting and getting to know new people. Compassion, care, and kindness for others would supersede "Getting someone to be with us."

And we would never try to control another person. We wouldn't put others on a pedestal, nor would we set them below us. We would remember that on the spiritual path, the purpose of any relationship is to wake up and get to know ourselves and our lover, thoroughly, without judgment or pride.

On the spiritual path, we enter into a shared union where we cherish and give to each other, expanding our ability to love unconditionally. We would accept that the process could be awkward, unpredictable, challenging and surprising. Ultimately, we would become friends with ourselves and give up demanding that the universe provide us with a lover. We would become open to meeting a special person with whom to share this journey of awakening.

"Like the grasses showing tender faces to each other, thus should we do also, for this was the wish of the Grandfathers of the world."
Black Elk, Native American

We Call A Halt

from the United Nations Environmental Sabbath Program

We who have lost our sense and our senses,
Our touch, our smell, our vision of who we are,
We who frantically force and press all things
Without rest for our body or spirit
Hurting our earth and injuring ourselves:
We call a halt.

We want to rest.
We need to rest and allow the earth to rest.
We need to reflect
And to rediscover the mystery that lives in us,
That is the ground of every unique expression of life,
The source of the fascination that calls all things to
communion.

We declare a Sabbath,
A space of quiet,
For simply being and letting be,
For recovering the great, forgotten truths,
For learning how to live again.

*"When all the trees have been cut down, when all the animals
have been hunted, when all the waters are polluted, when all the
air is unsafe to breathe, only then will you discover that you cannot
eat money." Cree Prophecy, Native American*

13

Creating A New Way Of Life *by Shakti Gawain*

WE ARE LIVING IN an exciting and powerful time. On the deepest level of consciousness, a radical spiritual transformation is taking place. On a worldwide level, we are being challenged to let go of our present way of life and create an entirely new one. We are, in fact, in the process of releasing our old world and building a new world in its place.

The change begins with each individual, but as more and more individuals are being transformed, the mass consciousness is increasingly affected, and the results will be manifested in the world around us.

The old world was based on an external focus. We had come to believe that the material world was the only reality. Thus, feeling essentially lost, empty, and alone, we have continually attempted to find happiness through addiction to external things such as money, material possessions, relationships, work, fame, food or drugs.

Today, as we begin to remember our fundamental spiritual connection, we can look within for the source of our satisfaction, joy and fulfillment. The new world is being built as we open to the higher power of the universe and consciously allow that creative energy to move through us. As each of us connects with our spiritual awareness, we learn that the creative power of the universe is within us. We also learn that we can create our own reality and take responsibility for doing so.

The new world is based on trust of the universe within us. We recognize that the creative intelligence and energy of the universe is the fundamental source of everything. Once we connect with this and surrender to it, everything is ours. Emptiness is filled from the inside.

The obvious question arises: "How can we contact this power, or gain access to it?" The knowingness that resides in each of us can be accessed through what we call our intuition. By learning to contact, listen to, and act on our intuition, we can directly connect to the higher power of the universe and allow it to become our guiding force.

"The intuitive mind is a sacred gift and the rational mind a faithful servant. We have created a society that honors the servant and has forgotten the gift." Albert Einstein

We Are Travelers On A Cosmic Journey

by Deepak Chopra

WE ARE TRAVELERS on a cosmic journey—stardust, swirling and dancing in the eddies and whirlpools of infinity. Life is eternal, but the expressions of life are ephemeral, momentary and transient. Gautama Buddha, the founder of Buddhism, once said:

> "This existence of ours is as transient as autumn clouds.
> To watch the birth and death of beings is like looking
> At the movements of a dance.
> A lifetime is like a flash of lightning in the sky,
> Rushing by like a torrent down a steep mountain."

We have stopped for a moment to encounter each other, to meet, to love, to share.

This is a precious moment, but it is transient. It is a little parenthesis in eternity. If we share with caring, lightheartedness, and love, we will create abundance and joy for each other and then this moment will have been worthwhile.

"What is life? It is the flash of a firefly in the night. It is the breath of a buffalo in the wintertime. It is the little shadow which runs across the grass and loses itself in the sunset." Crowfoot, Native American

15

Where Is God For The Lutheran Girl Who Turned To Zen *by Karen Sunna*

As a young girl I always wondered where God was. Once I went and sat in the Lutheran church to see if he was there, but all that happened was that the pastor came and invited me to his office to ask why my father never came to church, sort of like church social work. I never could find God in the hymns or the prayers or anything. Finally I gave up and stopped going to church.

Later, when I was in graduate school I found out that there is a way to sit down on the ground and fold my legs and arms together in a way that my parents never taught me. I sat that way for a long time. At last I came to realize that no matter where I was sitting I was always in the palm of the hand that we call God, or Buddha, or Allah, or whatever. That was a big discovery.

To experience this it was important to have no agenda. Ordinarily, I have a big head jumping full of beta waves. Worry is my best friend and worst enemy. Over time, I went to see a number of psychotherapists, even became one myself and did that as my work for years. It was reassuring, but it didn't touch the deep worry.

I began to realize that freedom meant letting go, putting down my burden, but I could never do it. Then I learned by doing psychotherapy that the best way to get over neurotic patterns is to just get good and tired of them. Sometimes the burdens drop then and a moment of space appears. Sometimes there are stretches of time when everything is fresh at every moment; everything encountered is bright and shiny. When I am doing the same dishes in the same kitchen as yesterday, it's all new and fully alive.

This is the way I want to live. This is living in the palm of the Buddhas, walking with Jesus, dancing with Shiva.

"You can enter yoga, or the path of yoga, only when you are totally frustrated with your own mind as it is. If you are still hoping that you can gain something through your mind, yoga isn't for you."
OSHO

16

Green Cheese *by John Mundahl*

When we're children, we say:

"For centuries people thought the moon was made of
green cheese.
Then the astronauts found out that the moon is really a
big hard rock.
That's what happens when you leave it out."
And we laugh.

Then we grow older and fall in love and say:

"Come, my love, the moon is full.
Lie with me tonight. Don't go.
See the meadow down below with moonlight all aglow."
And we laugh.

Then we grow old and our life comes to an end and we
say:

"So! The whole time it was really You!
Not the moon or green cheese!
It was really You, the light behind the moon, that was
real!"
And we laugh.

*"Hidden behind My magic veil of shows, I am not seen by all. I
am not known, the unborn and changeless, to all the idle world."
From the Bhagavad-Gita*

Earth, Teach Me *A Ute Prayer, Native American*

Earth teach me quiet—as the grasses are still with new light.

Earth teach me suffering—as old stones suffer with memory.

Earth teach me humility—as blossoms are humble with beginning.

Earth teach me caring—as mothers nurture their young.

Earth teach me courage—as the tree that stands alone.

Earth teach me limitation—as the ant that crawls on the ground.

Earth teach me freedom—as the eagle that soars in the sky.

Earth teach me acceptance—as the leaves that die each fall.

Earth teach me renewal—as the seed that rises in the spring.

Earth teach me to forget myself—as melted snow forgets its life.

Earth teach me to remember kindness—as dry fields weep with rain.

"I only went out for a walk but decided to stay out until sundown, for going out, I found, was really going in." John Muir

A New Dream *by Don Miguel Ruiz*

I WANT YOU TO forget everything you have learned in your whole life. This is the beginning of a new understanding, a new dream. The dream you are living is your creation. It is your perception of reality that you can change at any time. You have the power to create hell, and you have the power to create heaven. Why not dream a different dream? Why not use your mind, your imagination, and your emotions to dream heaven?

Just use your imagination and a tremendous thing will happen. Imagine that you have the ability to see the world with different eyes, whenever you choose, and each time you open your eyes, you see the world around you in a different way. Close your eyes now, and then open them and look outside. What you will see is love coming out of the trees, love coming out of the sky, love coming out of the light. This is the state of bliss.

"There's only one reason why you're not experiencing bliss at this present moment, and it's because you're thinking or focusing on what you don't have." Anthony DeMello

The Final Analysis

by Mother Teresa, original version by Kent M. Keith.

People are often unreasonable, illogical and self-centered;
Forgive them anyway.
If you are kind, people may accuse you of selfish, ulterior motives;
Be kind anyway.
If you are successful, you will win some false friends and some true enemies;
Succeed anyway.
If you are honest and frank, people may cheat you;
Be honest and frank anyway.
What you spend years building, someone may destroy overnight;
Build anyway.
If you find serenity and happiness, they may be jealous;
Be happy anyway.
The good you do today, people will often forget tomorrow;
Do good anyway.
Give the world the best you have, and it may never be enough;
Give the world the best you've got anyway.
You see, in the final analysis, it is all between you and God;
It was never between you and them anyway.

"Anyone who proposes to do good must not expect people to roll stones out of the way, but must accept his or her lot calmly, even if they roll a few more upon it." Albert Schweitzer

20

The Invitation *by Oriah Mountain Dreamer*

It doesn't interest me what you do for a living. I want to know what you ache for, and if you dare to dream of meeting your heart's longing.

It doesn't interest me how old you are. I want to know if you will risk looking like a fool for love, for your dream, for the adventure of being alive.

It doesn't interest me what planets are squaring your moon. I want to know if you have touched the center of your own sorrow, if you have been opened by life's betrayals or have become shriveled and closed from fear of further pain.

I want to know if you can sit with pain, mine or your own, without moving to hide it or fade it or fix it. I want to know if you can be with joy, mine or your own, if you can dance with wildness and let the ecstasy fill you to the tips of your fingers and toes without cautioning us to be careful, to be realistic, to remember the limitations of being human.

It doesn't interest me if the story you are telling me is true. I want to know if you can disappoint another to be true to yourself, if you can bear the accusation of betrayal and not betray your own soul, if you can be faithless and therefore trustworthy. I want to know if you can see Beauty even when it's not pretty, every day. And if you can source your own life from its presence. I want to know if you can live with failure, yours and mine, and still stand on the edge of the lake and shout to the silver of the full moon, "Yes."

It doesn't interest me to know where you live or how much money you have. I want to know if you can get up after the night of grief and despair weary and bruised to the bone and do what needs to be done to feed the children.

It doesn't interest me who you know or how you came to be here. I want to know if you will stand in the center of the fire with me and not shrink back. It doesn't interest me where or what or with whom you have studied. I want to know what sustains you from the inside when all else falls away. I want to know if you can be alone with yourself and if you truly like the company you keep in the empty moments.

"I came to yoga class to heal my body and I found myself instead."
Anonymous

The Super Bowl Yogi *by John Mundahl*

When I first started yoga
There was a man who came to my class.
He seldom spoke, but he wasn't unkind.
We would exchange smiles
And set up our yoga mats next to each other.
We were the only men in class.

I was learning the postures, so I liked to watch him.
He was older than me, but limber and strong,
And moved with grace,
Full of joy,
From one posture to the next…
    Never straining,
    His breath soft and easy,
    Drawn out in a natural way,
    Smooth and long,
    In beautiful rhythm
    With his body.
He kept his eyes closed and there was a smile of love
On his face from someplace deep inside him
That I wanted to discover for myself.

So one cold winter day,
I broke the silence between us.
    "Charlie," I asked. "Did you watch the Super Bowl?"
    "27-23 Pittsburgh," he said. "Big Ben had quite a
    day."
That was all he said.
Then he casually walked out the door
Into the frigid Minnesota winter
With no jacket,
No hat,

And no gloves.
Whew! I thought.
I don't have to give up football!

"What is the path?" Someone asked the Zen Master, Nan-sen.
"Everyday life is the path," he answered.

Sir, What Do You And Your Monks Practice?

By Thich Nhat Hanh

IN BUDDHISM, OUR EFFORT is to practice mindfulness in each moment…to know what is going on within and all around us. Once someone asked the Buddha,

"Sir, what do you and your monks practice?"

"We sit, we walk, and we eat," the Buddha replied.

"But sir," the questioner continued. "Everyone sits, walks, and eats."

"Yes," the Buddha said, "But when we sit, we *know* we are sitting.

When we walk, we *know* we are walking. When we eat, we *know* we are eating."

Most of the time we are lost in the past or carried away by future projects and concerns. When our mindfulness touches the present moment, we can see and listen deeply. The fruits are always understanding, acceptance, love and the desire to relieve suffering and bring joy. When our beautiful child comes up to us and smiles, we are completely there for her.

"In walking, just walk. In sitting, just sit. Above all, don't wobble." Yun-men

The Day I Discovered The Meaning Of Love

by Helen Keller

I REMEMBER THE MORNING that I first asked the meaning of the word, "love." Miss Sullivan put her arm gently around me and spelled into my hand,

"I love Helen."

"But what is love?" I asked.

She drew me closer to her and said,

"It's here," pointing to my heart, whose beats I was conscious of for the first time. Her words puzzled me because I didn't then understand anything unless I touched it.

"Is love the sweetness of flowers?" I asked.

"No," she said.

"Is it the warmth of the sun?"

"No," she said, and I was greatly disappointed. Then she touched my forehead and spelled the word, "Think," and in a flash I knew that some words described the process that was going on inside my head. This was my first conscious perception of an abstract idea.

For a long time I tried to understand the meaning of "love" in light of this new idea. One day it rained and then it stopped and the sun came out.

"Is this love?" I asked.

"You can't touch the clouds," Miss Sullivan said, "But you can feel the rain and know how glad the flowers and earth are to have it after a hot day. You can't touch love, either, but you can feel the sweetness that it pours into everything. Without love you wouldn't be happy or want to play."

The beautiful truth burst into my mind and I felt there were invisible lines stretched between my spirit and the spirits of others.

"Unity is the reality. Separateness the illusion. The nearer we come to reality, the nearer we come to unity of heart. Sympathy, compassion, kindness are modes of this unity of heart, whereby we rejoice with those who rejoice and weep with those who weep."
The Yoga Sutras of Patanjali

A Grieving Woman and the Mustard Seed

a Buddhist parable

KISA GOTAMI'S DAUGHTER HAD DIED and she was in agony over the loss. She had heard that the Buddha was capable of miracles and she went to him, begging for her daughter to be brought back to life. The Buddha felt great compassion for the poor woman and promised he would help her—but only if she could bring him some mustard seed from a home that had known no sorrow.

Filled with hope, Kisa set out on her search. She knew that mustard seed was a common spice and surely every home in the village had some. But as she knocked on every door, she heard one sad story after another.

"Oh, we lost Grandfather last year."

"My son was born with a clubfoot and can't walk."

"My mother suffers from palsy and is near death."

"I lost two daughters in childbirth and have just miscarried again."

Everywhere she went, the story was the same: sorrow, loss and grief marked every home.

Soon Kisa realized that suffering was universal. No human on earth could escape sorrow and loss. She returned to the Buddha and asked,

"What do I do now?"

Buddha's teaching for coping with universal suffering touched her heart and she became one of his earliest and most devoted followers.

"Yoga teaches us to cure what need not be endured and endure what cannot be cured." B.K.S. Iyengar

Are Your Potatoes Heavy? *Author unknown.*

A TEACHER ONCE TOLD each of her students to bring a clear plastic bag and a sack of potatoes to school. For every person they refused to forgive in their life, the students had to choose a potato, write a name and date on it, and put the potato in the plastic bag. Some of their bags were quite heavy.

They were then told to carry this bag with them everywhere for one week, putting it beside their bed at night, on the car seat when driving, next to their desk at school.

The hassle of lugging this around with them made it clear what a weight they were carrying spiritually, and how they had to pay attention all the time so they wouldn't leave the bag in embarrassing places. Naturally the condition of the potatoes deteriorated to a nasty smelly slime.

This is a great metaphor for the price we pay for holding on to our pain and heavy negativity. Too often we think of forgiveness as a gift to the other person and it clearly is a gift for ourselves.

"If you are irritated by every rub, how will you ever be polished?"
Rumi

It's Simple *author unknown*

O NCE A MAN was having a conversation with the Lord.

"Lord, I would like to know what Heaven and Hell are like," he said.

The Lord led the man to two doors. He opened one of the doors and the man looked in. In the middle of the room was a large round table. In the middle of the table was a large pot of stew, which smelled delicious and made the man's mouth water. But the people sitting around the table were thin and sickly. They appeared famished. They were holding spoons with long handles that were strapped to their arms and each found it possible to reach into the pot of stew and take a spoonful, but because the handle was longer than their arms, they couldn't get the spoons back into their mouths. The man shuddered at the sight of their misery and suffering.

"You have seen hell," the Lord said.

Then they went to the next room and opened the door. It was exactly the same as the first one. There was the large round table with the large pot of stew which made the man's mouth water. The people had the same long-handled spoons, but here the people were well nourished and plump, laughing and talking.

"I don't understand," the man said.

"It's simple," the Lord said. "In this place the people have learned to feed one another."

"If we have no peace, it is because we have forgotten we belong to each other." Mother Teresa

An Evening Darshan *by John Mundahl*

One winter, when the farm lay soft and white,
Caught off guard by early snow,
A deer stood outside my window
Looking in to see if I was there.
I knew her. I had fed her last year
And knew her by the ear that flopped to one side.
"Back so soon?" I said, "Or just too lazy to dig in snow
For evening meal? No matter!"
And I rose to fetch the corn from the shed where it lay drying.

She was waiting for me,
Out by the tree where I had fed her last year.
I put the yellow cobs down and left
And went inside to watch her feed.
But she walked away and I was puzzled.
Surely she was hungry, her sunken sides told me so.
Then I watched her beat the snow with front hoof
Until her spring fawn appeared, grown now, of course.

But he was sick or something and could barely walk,
Let alone feed himself.
Then I saw the little one had been shot, during the fall
Hunt, and she had brought him to the corn to feed.
She let him have his fill, watching as he ate.
At last she sighed, her own hunger now too much,
And she pushed her nose into the snow and ate what was left.

The little one limped away, full for the moment.
A long winter lay ahead for him. Too long, I feared.
He would never make it,

Though I kept the thought tucked to myself.
When she was finished eating, she walked up to my
Window again and held her pose, as if in thanks,
Knowing how much I loved to see her.
I pressed my palms together in simple prayer position
And thanked her for her darshan.
Then she hurried off, a worried look on her face,
Toward the distant tree line where her little one stood
Waiting, shivering, I thought, in the evening chill.

"Yoga gives. It does not take from the world. It adds gentleness to the general good." Anonymous

Beyond Even The Solid Me *by Nancy Ann James*

A NOTED ZEN MASTER is often quoted: "To study Buddhism is to study the self, to learn the self is to forget the self." Although I had always been somewhat shy and self-conscious, finally, little by little, that self-consciousness was falling away. I was finding the solid me that had been there all along, underneath the doubter and the actor—the performer—the conditioned good girl. And one day, I went beyond even the solid me.

…It happens during a seven-day Zen meditation session, on the fourth day. A lot of things have led up to it, but shortly after seating myself at 5 a.m. in the dimly lit zendo, facing the wall, it hits me that I have no problems whatsoever. "Only the small self has problems" are the words that float into my consciousness. Whereas I, or this collection of cells known as Nancy, have somehow entered the realm of the big Self.

The feeling is of complete joy and appreciation. When another sitter comes in late and sits down next to me, I gaze at his bare foot sitting on his left thigh and almost bend down to kiss it, it is so beautiful. It's a foot just being a foot. In the chanting during a service after several sittings, the words I'm chanting and have chanted many times before, suddenly make total sense. Particularly clear is the line, accompanied by a gentle ring of the bell, "And the mind is no hindrance."

My mind suddenly is no hindrance whatsoever—not getting in the way as it usually does. It's as clear as the bell. Walking outside after breakfast, I wonder how I 'm going to be able to explain to anyone how, walking around the block at 7:30 in the morning on a June day in southeast Minneapolis, I'm the happiest I have ever been.

Seeing an old lady out sweeping her front steps, I want to go hug her, she's so completely—what? Just being herself. I restrain myself and call out to her something about the beautiful morning. Seeing lots of students and teachers walking fast and bicycling toward the university, their heads down, I want to shout something startling that will wake them up. Hearing a distant sound of a fire engine, I can only think: "That poor person with the fire thinks they have a problem. But only the small self has problems."

If only everyone could live in the big Self .

"When we find delight within ourselves and feel inner joy and pure contentment, there is nothing left to be done." The Bhagavad-Gita

29

He Is The Yogi *from the Bhagavad-Gita*

"The sovereign soul of him who lives self-governed
And at peace is centered in himself,
Taking alike pleasure and pain,
Heat and cold, glory and shame.
He is the yogi,
Glad with joy of love and truth,
Dwelling apart upon a peak, with senses subjugate,
Whereto the clod, the rock, the glistering gold show all
as one.
By this sign he is known:
Being of equal grace to comrades, friends, chance-comers,
Strangers, lovers, enemies, aliens and kinsmen—
Loving all alike, evil or good.
Sequestered should he sit, steadfastly meditating,
Solitary, his thoughts controlled,
His passions laid away, quit of belongings.
There, setting hard his mind upon The One,
Restraining heart and senses, silent, calm,
Let him accomplish Yoga and achieve pureness of soul."

30

Our First Play Date *by John Mundahl*

> Do you remember our first play date?
> You promised to meet me in the meadow
> Where the river bends toward the cottonwood trees.
> Remember?
> I said Saturday would work fine for me,
> And you said,
> "Saturday?
> Why not now?
> Here I am!
> Now!"
> And you tickled my toes
> And I couldn't stop laughing.

"Yoga takes you into the present moment, the only place where life exists." Anonymous

Yoga Has Taught Me Much *by Elizabeth Anderson*

Yoga has taught me much. Yoga has taught me that each morning I wake up to my own mind, not to the world the way it actually is. How can I understand others at all, then, except by who or what I think they are, or who or what I think they should be? I think we should give up the notion that we can ever completely understand the mystery of another, or that we need to. We should simply give them space, space to just be, and drop the idea that they are people who need fixing by me. When they speak, we should just listen, and feel no need to respond. When we speak, we should speak from the heart.

"Out beyond the ideas of wrong doing and right doing, there is a field. I'll meet you there." Rumi

It Felt Love *by Hafiz*

> How
> Did the rose
> Ever open its heart
>
> And give to this world
> All its
> Beauty?
>
> It felt the encouragement of light
> Against its
> Being,
>
> Otherwise,
> We all remain
> Too
> Frightened.

"And the day came when the risk it took to remain tight inside the bud was more painful than the risk it took to blossom." Anais Nin

A Blessing *by James Wright*

Just off the highway to Rochester, Minnesota,
Twilight bounds softly forth on the grass.
And the eyes of those two Indian ponies
Darken with kindness.
They have come gladly out of the willows
To welcome my friend and me.
We step over the barbed wire into the pasture
Where they have been grazing all day, alone.
They ripple tensely; they can hardly contain their happiness
That we have come.
They bow shyly as wet swans. They love each other.
There is no loneliness like theirs.
At home once more,
They begin munching the young tufts of spring in the darkness.
I would like to hold the slenderer one in my arms.
For she has walked over to me
And nuzzled my left hand.
She is black and white,
Her main falls wild on her forehead,
And the light breeze moves me to caress her long ear
That is delicate as the skin over a girl's wrist.
Suddenly I realize
That if I stepped out of my body I would break
Into blossom.

"Angels whisper to those who go for a walk." Stephen Wright

A Lotus For You, A Buddha To Be

by Thich Nhat Hanh

THE WORD "BUDDHA" comes from the root *buddh*, which means to wake up. A Buddha is someone who is awake. When Buddhists greet one another, we hold our palms together like a lotus flower, breathe in and out mindfully, bow, and say silently,

"A lotus for you, a Buddha to be."

This kind of greeting produces two Buddhas at the same time. We acknowledge the seeds of awakening, Buddhahood, that are within the other person, whatever his or her age or status. And we practice mindful breathing to touch the seed of Buddhahood within ourselves.

"Let us always meet each other with a smile, for the smile is the beginning of love." Mother Teresa

The Man Who Was Going To America

by Swami Kripalu

ONCE THERE WAS a well-known saint in India named Swami Ram Tirtha. He lived during the time of Swami Vivikananda. He was truly a non-attached mahatma. He decided to visit America, but before he left India, a man came up to him and asked,

"Are you really going to America?"

"Yes," he said.

"Please write to me and tell me when you're returning, as I would like to see you then."

"That's fine," Swami Ram Tirtha said.

Swami Ram Tirtha left for America, just as he had planned, and stayed a long time and created many devotees. When he returned to India, the same man found him.

"You're back from America now?" The man asked.

"Yes," Swami Ram Tirtha said.

"I'm also thinking of going to America," the man said. "How expensive is it?"

"There's no expense at all," Swami Ram Tirtha said.

"But I'm not a swami like you," the man said. "No one will give me food, money and passage. How can I go to America without money?"

"Brother," Swami Ram Tirtha said. "You're just *thinking* about going to America, so there's no expense involved. The expense comes only when you go there."

It's the same on the spiritual path. As long as we only think about going to God, there's no expense involved. The expense comes only when we decide to make the journey.

"In a world where death is the hunter, my friend, there is no time for regrets or doubts. There is only time for decisions." Carlos Castaneda

The Eyes Of Rumi *by John Mundahl*

I met a saint at Walmart once.
I was standing in line waiting to check out.
An elderly woman was behind the register.
 "You should be home," I thought,
 "Not standing on your feet all day."
But then I watched her greet everyone:
 Man or woman,
 Adult or child,
 Young or old,
 Clean or dirty,
 Crabby or kind,
 Rushed or patient,
 Angry or calm,
 Black or white,
 Tattoos,
 Spiked hair,
 Mohawks,
 Or bald…
None of it mattered to her.
She truly greeted each person with eyes of love,
Including me.
I never forgot her
And I still see her face
On long days when I need a blessing.

"Forgive us for every face we cannot look upon with joy."
Frederick Buechner

Awareness And The Mind *by Dr. David Frawley*

BEHIND CHANGING mental fluctuations is a constant awareness, an unbroken sense of self or being, an ongoing ability to observe, witness and perceive. Though the contents of the mind constantly shift, like clouds in the sky, there is ongoing continuity to our consciousness, like the purity of space, through which we can observe these with detachment. Therefore the mind itself is not awareness. It is the instrument that awareness works through, like a computer a person works with.

Awareness, unlike the mind, has no form, function or movement. It is not located in time and space but stands apart as their witness. It is not affected by action and remains free of good and bad results. To know this awareness, we must learn to go beyond the mind, which means to disengage from its involvements. This is our real work as human beings and the essence of the spiritual path, whatever form of it we choose to follow. As long as we are in the sphere of the mind, we are dominated by the external and cannot know the inner reality.

True awareness is Pure Consciousness beyond the mental field. Our ordinary awareness is conditioned within the mental field. Only because the light of pure awareness is reflected onto the mental field does the mind appear to be conscious. The mind itself, therefore, is not aware, intelligent or self-luminous. It works through the reflection of a greater light, a greater consciousness in which alone is understanding and freedom. We must learn to seek that pure light beyond the mind.

"One morning at the end of my practices, I turned my eyes upward toward the middle of my forehead and my mind dissolved into joy. It was overwhelming." Anonymous

The Journey Of Transformation *by Yogi Amrit Desai*

The journey of transformation begins with inward focus.
Meditative awareness harmonizes unconscious forces,
Restless mind and emotional conflicts.

Mindful meditative awareness transports you to another dimension,
Where you experience the unifying power of the spirit.
It leads you to a sacred space in the cave of your heart,
Where you can return again and again,
To regain the protective power of the Divine
That is always present in you.

As you enter this sacred space,
Leave your ego mind outside,
And invite the witness inside.
The witness is like a black hole;
Whatever you bring to it
Disappears into the void of nothingness,
Leaving nothing for you to do.

The most beautiful part of the witness
Is that you have no obligation
To process anything, to control anything, to expect anything.
Simply be in it.

"The world is a busy place that can't afford to give you the peace you are looking for because peace is not one of its products. If you continue to externalize your mind, then you will reap its diminishing returns." Swami Rama

I'm Back Now *by John Mundahl*

Yesterday morning I got up
And read the message I had written to myself
On the bathroom mirror:
    "Be kind today. Everyone is suffering."
But then on my way to work
Someone cut me off on the freeway and I got angry.
I had a long day at work, too.
    The air inside our building was dead and stale.
    My co-workers were stressed.
    I didn't get everything done that I needed to.
    The traffic was bad going home
    And I arrived home tired and hungry.

After supper I took a long walk in the park.
I tried to remember how I was connected to all things,
But I didn't feel connected to anything.
Then my small daughter softly took my hand.
    "Daddy," she asked, looking up at me, "Do you love
    me?"
    I was startled.
    "Of course I do, sweetie. Why?"
    "Because you were gone just now and I didn't know
    where you were and I got scared."
I reached down then and picked her up and swung her
around in the air and we both burst into laughter.
    "I'm back now," I said. "I'm back."

"A disturbed mind is always someplace else." Yogi Amrit Desai

A Meditation On Kindness *by Charlotte Kasl*

*Y*OU CAN IMAGINE *this or remember to do it when you are in a crowd:*

When you are in a crowd, look around at all the different people. Notice their clothes, faces, and hair sizes. Look at their gestures and movements, noticing if they are loose, stiff, or free. Just take it in, without judgment, as if you were looking at a garden of people.

Then see them all as energy fields, the same as you. Just energy. As you continue watching, think to yourself: Every person here has had to live every day of their lives, just like me. They have had to get up every day, decide what to wear, face loss, success, hurt, and shame, just like me. Everyone fell down while learning to walk, everyone probably felt anxious the first time they kissed, just like me. Each person has a story to tell. Some of the chapters are heroic. Some of them are about loss, some about fear, some about achievement or joy, just like my story. Then continue to think of them as energy, conceived as an egg and sperm, just like you.

When you say good-bye to someone or decide not to see them again, remember you are a moment in their story. Make it a story that doesn't leave a scar.

"Feelings are everywhere. Be gentle." J. Masai

That Is The Glory Of The Mystic *by Annie Besant*

A ND THINK WHAT IT MEANS if God to you is no longer a name but a life. That is the glory of the mystic, that is the joy of the one who knows. Wherever you go you see Him shining. You look at the wonder of nature spreading out before you and in the whole of that manifested beauty, as in the tiniest fragment, you see it all irradiated by the perfect beauty that is God. You see Him in the blue of the sky or ocean. You hear Him singing in every bird. You see Him smiling in every flower. And most of all, you see Him in the heart and in the intellect and in the love of men, women and children. You see Him in the righteousness of the most holy and you see Him hiding in the heart of the basest, illuminating it now and then with some touch of human love, which is the nearest of all things to God, whose very nature is love and bliss.

"Accustomed long to contemplating Love and Compassion, I have forgotten all difference between myself and others." Milarepa, Tibetan yogi.

The Beginning of Freedom *by Eckhart Tolle*

The beginning of freedom
Is the realization that you are not your mind,
The thinker.
Knowing this enables you to observe the entity.

The moment you start watching the thinker,
A higher level of consciousness becomes activated.
You then begin to realize
That there is a vast realm of intelligence beyond thought,
That thought is only a tiny aspect of that intelligence.

You also realize that all the things that truly matter:
Beauty, love, creativity, joy, inner peace,
Arise from beyond the mind.
You begin to awaken.

"I was so full of sleep that I left the true way." Dante

43

The Sermon Of Saint Francis To The Birds

ONE DAY as St. Francis was going he saw on some trees by the wayside a great multitude of birds. St. Francis was much surprised and said to his companions,

"Wait for me here while I go and preach to my little sisters the birds."

And he entered into the field and began to preach to the birds which were on the ground, and those which were in the trees came round him and all listened while St. Francis preached to them and none flew away until they had attained his blessing.

"My little sisters the birds," he said, "ye owe much to God, your Creator, and ye ought to sing his praise at all times and in all places, because he has given you liberty to fly about into all places. And though ye neither spin now sew, he has given you a twofold and a threefold clothing for yourselves and your offspring. Two of all your species he sent into the Ark with Noah that you might not be lost to the world; and he feeds you though ye neither sow nor reap.

He has given you fountains and rivers to quench your thirst, mountains and valleys in which to take refuge, and trees in which to build your nests. So the Creator loves you very much, having thus favored you with such bounties. Beware my little sisters of the sin of ingratitude and study always to give praise to God."

After he had said these words, all the birds began to open their beaks, to stretch their necks, to spread their wings, and reverently bow their heads to the ground. And the Saint rejoiced with them and finished his sermon and made the sign of the cross and the birds flew away.

"God dwells in the heart of all being, Arjuna, thy God dwells in thy heart, and His power of wonder moves all things...puppets in a play of shadows...whirling them onward on the stream of time." From the Bhagavad-Gita

The Dancer And The Starfish *author unknown*

ONCE UPON A TIME there was a wise man who used to go to the ocean to do his writing. He had a habit of walking on the beach before he began his work. One day he was walking along the shore. As he looked down the beach, he saw a person moving like a dancer. He smiled to himself to think of someone who would dance on this morning. So he began to walk faster to catch up. As he got closer, he saw it was a young man and the young man wasn't dancing, but instead he was reaching down to the shore, picking up something and gently throwing it into the ocean. As he got closer he called out,

"Good morning! What are you doing?" The young man paused, looked up and replied, "Throwing starfish into the ocean."

"Why are you throwing starfish into the ocean?"

"The sun is up and the tide is going out and if I don't throw them in they'll die."

"But, young man, there are miles and miles of beach and starfish all along it. You can't possibly make a difference!"

The young man listened politely. Then he bent down, picked up another starfish and threw it into the sea past the breaking waves and said,

"It made a difference to that one."

"In this life we cannot do great things. We can only do small things with great love." Mother Teresa

The God Who Only Knows Four Words *by Hafiz*

Every
Child
Has known God,
Not the God of names,
Not the God of don't,
Not the God who ever does
Anything weird,
But the God who only knows four words
And keeps repeating them, saying:

"Come dance with Me."
Come
Dance.

"A sad saint is a sad saint." Paramahansa Yogananda

The Cider Stand *by John Mundahl*

Which road was it that I took
Just before the Woodstock winter
When I stumbled half surprised
Upon the hidden cider stand?
Perhaps just off the Jersey Parkway
Or north beyond the Catskills
Driving to someplace I've long forgotten.

But tucked within a friendly wood,
On a road leafed with autumn,
Sat the stand with old man close.
He with apple cheeks
Quick to laugh at grumpy pumpkins.

"One cider, please," I said.
"Hot?"
"Please."

With two old hands flannelled tight,
He drew a steaming glass of cider.
I drank it sweet among the gourds and Indian corn,
Then turned to thank, but he was busy.

From a glance I sensed he was a happy man,
Wanting nothing more than his cider stand
And health to draw the juice for those who asked.
I felt that like his apples
He had placed his yesterdays into his cider press
And found the juice that streamed forth
Sweet,
Not bitter.

"Yoga changes you, not the world. It cultivates your viewpoint."
Anonymous

Heartprints *author unknown*

Whatever our hands touch,
We leave fingerprints,
On walls, on furniture,
On doorknobs, dishes, books.
There's no escape.
As we touch we leave our identity.

Wherever I go today
Help me leave heartprints.
Heartprints of compassion,
Of understanding and love.

Heartprints of kindness
And genuine concern.
May my heart touch a lonely neighbor,
Or a runaway daughter,
Or an anxious mother,
Or perhaps an aged grandfather.

Send me out today
To leave heartprints.
And if someone should say,
"I felt your touch,"
May they also sense the love
That is deep within my heart.

*"The eye never forgets what the heart has seen." Bantu Culture
Proverb*

48

This, Too, Shall Pass *by Maria Garcia*

YOGA HAS ALLOWED ME to slow down mentally. I was always rushing, rushing, rushing. My mind was always someplace else and I was missing it all…the play of light on the trees, a spider web wet with dew, the subtle messages from within. More and more now I can simply be with what is. I'm happier and healthier and I'm a better mother to my children. When they spill the milk or come to me crying my first thought now is: This, too, shall pass. More and more everything is becoming a show to me, a show in Technicolor.

"Everything passes, and what remains of former times, what remains of life, is the spiritual. In everything we do, the claim of the Absolute is unchanging." Paul Klee

The Charity Loved By The Lord *by Swami Kripalu*

The Lord secretly nourishes the sun and the moon with
light.
He secretly fills the earth with food.
He secretly fills the clouds with water.

Yes, we can clearly see the sun, the moon, the light,
The earth, the food, the clouds, and the water,
But our eyes cannot see the Lord,
Or any part of His body, or even His shadow.

The Creator of the world is so great that He works in
silence.
Since we are His children,
Shouldn't our nature contain a bit of His charity?

The charity loved by the Lord has two wings:
Give Secretly, and, *Give and Forget.*
That is, as much as possible,
We should give without others knowing.

Pure charity is only that which we give with compassion
and religious feeling.
When a devotee offers pure charity with faith to God,
God feels tremendously content and merges with the
devotee,
Making him, or her, his own.

*"Love and compassion are necessities. Without them, humanity
cannot survive." The Dalai Lama*

The Promise *by John Mundahl*

One fall, as the trees were turning,
I walked with my daughter
Along a trail in the woods
Just to kick the leaves a bit
And watch the busy squirrels get ready for winter.
She was only four
And chatted more than the bluejays.
Every tree and stump along the matted path
Brought a new surprise.

Soon, though, she got tired;
The fresh air was too much,
So I picked her up
And put her on my shoulder.
        "Daddy," she said softly. "Promise me something?"
        "Sure," I said.
        "This shoulder is only for me."
        "I promise."
        "And you never break a promise, do you."
        "Never," I said.
Then she tucked her head under my chin and fell asleep.
The path led on past red maples and a beaver pond
And then back to the car,
But the little bundle on my shoulder never got heavy
And I kept the promise.

*"With all its sham, drudgery and broken dreams, it is still a
beautiful world. Be cheerful. Strive to be happy." Max Ehrman,
from Desiderate*

The Debt Of Karma *by Yogi Amrit Desai*

Every soul is charged with an evolutionary mission
To realize its inborn divine potential.
Life is a perpetual therapeutic irritation.
It provides a compelling force to drive us
Toward the completion of our mission.
When we deny a painful experience,
It goes underground as a pending debt of unfinished
karma.
When you block pain, you may feel temporary relief,
But your karmic account is not closed.
The collection agency will present the lesson
Again and again, in various forms,
Through apparently unrelated events.
Every event that is not faced fully and consciously comes
back
As irritation, emotion, resistance or denial.
Habitual ways of reacting and reliving the same event
Perpetuate unconsciousness.
All lessons will be repeated until they are learned.
The debt of karma is paved in consciousness.

*"No sage ever made it to the other shore without getting
shipwrecked." Swami Rama*

A Higher Level of Healing *by Dr. David Frawley*

F OR MOST OF US, medical treatment begins when we fall ill. It is a form of disease treatment, a response to a condition that has already occurred. It aims at fixing something already broken. However, if medicine begins with the treatment of disease, it is a failure because the disease is already harming us. At this late state, radical and invasive methods may be required, like drugs or surgery, which have many side effects.

A higher level of healing is to eliminate diseases before they manifest, for which invasive methods like drugs or surgery are seldom necessary. To reach this stage we must consider the effects of our lifestyle, environment, work and psychological condition. We must cut off the wrong factors in our daily lives that make us vulnerable to disease.

To some extent, we are always sick because life itself is transient and unstable. There is always some disease attacking, particularly in changes of season or in the aging process. Each creature that is born must eventually die. Health is a matter of continual adjustment, like sailing a ship upon the sea. It cannot be permanently achieved and then forgotten, but is an ongoing concern.

"They must change often who would be constant in happiness."
Confucius

He Thinks He's Somebody *by John Mundahl*

He thinks because he dunks a basketball
That he's a special man,
That the world is his to do with as he pleases.

He thinks because he hits a baseball far
That he's a special man,
That the world is his to do with as he pleases.

He thinks because he hits a golf ball straight
That he's a special man,
That the world is his to do with as he pleases.

But,
What is the connection
Between
An extraordinary body
And an extraordinary soul?

Nothing.
Less than nothing.
Gandhi weighed 95 pounds
Yet he kicked the British out of India.

Go and see your neighbor.
Have lunch with him.
Get *his* autograph.
Get his jersey, too.
He mows his lawn each week
And puts his kids to bed on time.

"My son, greatness lies in one's character and not in worldly substances like gold or silver. If that is true, what is the difference between a seat of gold and a heap of dust? A diamond always remains a diamond, whether it's embedded in gold or silver or lost in mud." Lord Lakulish to Swami Kripalu

Now Is The Time *by Hafiz*

Now is the time to know
That all you do is sacred.

Now, why not consider
A lasting truce with yourself and God.

Now is the time to understand
That all your ideas of right and wrong
Were just a child's training wheels
To be laid aside
When you can finally live
With veracity
And love.

Hafiz is a divine envoy
Whom the Beloved
    Has written a holy message upon.

My dear, please tell me,
Why do you still
Throw sticks at your heart
And God?

What is it in that sweet voice inside
That incites you to fear?

Now is the time for the world to know
That every thought and action is sacred.

This is the time
For you to deeply compute the impossibility

That there is anything
But Grace.

Now is the season to know
That everything you do
Is sacred.

"Something sacred, that's it. We ought to be able to say that such and such a painting is as it is, with its capacity for power, because it is 'touched by God.'" Pablo Picasso

Know the Sweet Joy of Living in the Way

by the Buddha

Live in joy, in love, even among those who hate.
Live in joy, in health, even among the afflicted.
Live in joy, in peace, even among the troubled.
Look within. Be still, free from fear and attachment,
Know the sweet joy of living in the way.

There is no fire like greed, no crime like hatred,
No sorrow like hunger of heart, and no joy like the joy of freedom.
Health, contentment and trust are your greatest possessions,
And freedom your greatest joy.
Look within. Be still, free from fear and attachment.
Know the sweet joy of living in the way.

"To the mind that is still, the whole universe surrenders." Lieh Tzu

Final Advice *by John Mundahl*

When my father was dying we kept him home.
His wasn't dying from ill health,
Just old age and too much Norwegian food.
He was a man of few words, so he slept mostly.
When the end came,
My mother found me,
Straightened her apron,
And said,
"John. Your father wants to see you."
Well, I thought,
This is it,
His final advice.

I walked into his room and sat down next to his bed.
His eyes were closed and there was no breath,
And for a moment, I thought he was already gone.
But then he woke up, confused at first,
Like a visitor from another world.
When he recognized me,
He looked me squarely in the eye and said,
"Son, remember to feed the chickadees.
They like black sunflower seeds.
Buy the 25-pound bag. It's cheaper."
That was it.
He left then, a happy man, and I kept the feeders full.

*"Live like there's no tomorrow. Love like you've never lost. And
dance like no one's watching." Anonymous*

A Discourse On Love—*Metta Sutta (Suttanipata I)*

H E OR SHE WHO wants to attain peace should practice being upright, humble, and capable of using loving speech. He or she will know how to live simply and happily, with senses calmed, without being covetous and carried away by the emotions of the majority. Let him or her not do anything that will be disapproved of by the wise ones.

This is what he or she contemplates:

May everyone be happy and safe, and may their hearts be filled with joy.

May all living beings live in security and peace—beings who are frail or strong, tall or short, big or small, visible or not visible, near or far away, already born or yet to be born. May all of them dwell in perfect tranquility.

Let no one do harm to anyone. Let no one put the life of anyone in danger. Let no one, out of anger or ill will, wish anyone any harm.

Just as a mother loves and protects her only child at the risk of her own life, we should cultivate Boundless Love to offer to all living beings in the entire cosmos. We should let our boundless love pervade the whole universe, above, below and across. Our love will know no obstacles; our heart will be absolutely free from hatred and enmity. Whether standing or walking, sitting or lying, as long as we are awake, we should maintain this mindfulness of love in our own heart. This is the noblest way of living.

Free from wrong views, greed and sensual desires, living in beauty and realizing perfect understanding, those who practice boundless love will certainly transcend birth and death.

The Old Master Whips The Young Prince

by Swami Kripalu

O NCE THERE WAS AN old acharya, an old spiritual teacher. He was an exceptional saint and an exceptional teacher. He served the king of that area and the king respected him so much that he never disobeyed an order from this saint, even though he himself was the king.

The king had one son.

One day the king called the old master to his side and said,

"I'm getting old. The prince is ready to sit upon the throne. I'd like to have a coronation ceremony. Please plan this in keeping with the scriptures."

The acharya planned the ceremony with the help of others in the court, and when the festive day arrived, everyone in the kingdom celebrated. That morning the king and queen inspected the special clothes that the prince was to wear, along with the jewelry and ornaments.

"Everything is fine," the king said. "Bathe and dress the prince now for the ceremony."

But when the prince was only half dressed, he received a message from the acharya. The message said come at once to see me.

The prince was surprised. What could be so important that his teacher would call him now? The prince left immediately because he, too, never disobeyed an order from this great saint. Maybe Guruji wants to tell me something special, the young prince thought, since this is such an important day in my life.

The prince entered the acharya's room and bowed to him. Immediately the acharya took a whip off the wall and whipped him hard on his bare back! Then he did it four more times! He whipped him so hard there were marks and blood on his back.

The prince screamed with pain!

"Why is Guruji punishing me?" He asked himself. "Normally Guruji is gentle and explains everything to me! Today he's punishing me severely and yet saying nothing! I must have made some mistake!"

When the beating was over, the young prince stood up and looked into the face of his teacher. The old acharya's face was peaceful, totally balanced and calm, and full of compassion for the young prince.

The attendants rushed out to tell the king and soon the king and queen and many others arrived. Here it was, such a happy day, full of music and dancing, and yet the prince was being beaten? No one could understand this.

The prince left the room and everyone saw the marks and blood on his back. They saw the pain and hurt on his face and the tears in his eyes. They knew he had an innocent nature, yet no one dared say a word, not even the king. The old acharya was loved and respected so much that no one ever doubted the wisdom of his actions.

Everyone returned inside the palace and the great coronation ceremony continued. By the end of the day, the young prince had become the new king.

"Maharaja," the old acharya said to the young prince the next day. "Now you're the king, so I'll call you Maharaja. Now you must serve as final Judge on all matters in the kingdom. So I ask you to administer justice to me for the harsh beating I gave you yesterday."

The young king became silent.

"Why did you punish me?" He asked softly

"I saw the need for it," the old acharya said.

"Did I commit some wrong? Did I make a mistake?"

"No, you did nothing wrong."

"Then why did you punish me?"

"To teach you a lesson."

"What is the lesson?"

"You were born into the family of a king. You were raised with great love. You have never experienced physical punishment. Now you're the king and you must pass judgment on others. I wanted you to know the pain of physical punishment so that you don't rule too harshly. You must punish people with understanding."

The young king stood up and bowed to his teacher.

"Guruji," he said softly. "I know the horrible pain of the whip now and I won't be unjust to anyone."

"May you rule with compassion," the old acharya said, and then he left the room.

"The pain of others does not touch everyone. Those touched by the pain of others are God's messengers because God can comfort his suffering children through them." Swami Kripalu

I Am Already *by Danna Faulds*

One flow of
Energy and breath
Connects the full
Depth and breadth
Of consciousness.
There is nowhere to
Go but here, no time
But now, no why or
How or maybe…just
This knowing, simple
And complete, that I
Am already what I
Thought I had to seek.

"All you need for doing yoga is your body the way it is and your mind to say: 'You're fine. There's nothing that needs fixing before you can begin.'" Anonymous

60

Swami Rama and the Fire *by Swami Rama.*

ONCE I GOT RESTLESS in our monastery and began to think about living in the world rather than roaming in the mountains. My master walked in and told me to follow him. He led me to a deep cave in the mountains where donations over the centuries had piled up. I saw a huge, twelve-foot mount of gold, silver and jewels. I was transfixed by their allurement. My master, of course, knew well my liking for fine jewels.

Suddenly, I noticed that he was gone. I turned to the side of the cave and saw my master standing alone, completely enveloped in flames. The contrasting sights between the flames and the riches overwhelmed me.

"Make your choice!" My master called to me. "Either enter the world and take all those treasures, or else follow me into the fire!"

I stepped into the flames of my master. All my desires for the world and its allurements were burned to ashes that day.

"Nothing real can be threatened. Nothing unreal exists. Herein lies the peace of God." From A Course in Miracles

Pondering The Dharma *by John Mundahl*

Dharma
Means our duty,
Our natural purpose.
It's the dharma of the sun to shine.
It's the dharma of a cat to chase mice.
It's the dharma of human beings to learn to love.

Love *is* the work of the soul.
Love *is* the joy beyond all form.

So let us bury the grudge and all the sorrows
And do our soul work together,
Clumsy though our steps may be.

God didn't create this park so we could just play.

But what do I know?
Listen to Rumi:
*"Every second that unravels far from love
Is a source of shame before the Lord."*

Yoga, My Dad, And Me *by Rebecca Mundahl*

When I was a child,
I did yoga postures with my dad.
My favorite posture was simply to run
And jump on him whenever I could.
He just laughed!
And I learned that yoga was patient and kind.

When I became a teenager,
I left yoga to hang out with my friends.
I ate food that made me sick
And stayed up late and learned to drive.
My dad just kept doing the headstand
And making his own yogurt
And I learned that yoga was tolerant and accepting.

Now I'm a young woman,
And going to yoga class is as normal as breathing.
I'm seldom sick.
I laugh more than I cry.
I like myself when I look in the mirror,
Usually,
And I've learned that yoga is a way of life.

*"I do yoga with my children. We turn the postures into a game.
Then afterwards we sit in silence for a few minutes. Sometimes the
roles drop, me as parent, they as children, and I know for certain
that we are souls who have come together again." Anonymous*

A Practice for the New Millennium

by the Dalai Lama

Spend 5 minutes at the beginning of each day remembering we all want the same things…to be happy and to be loved, and we are all connected to one another.

Spend 5 minutes breathing in, cherishing yourself, and breathing out, cherishing others. If you think about people you have difficulty cherishing, extend your cherishing to them anyway.

During the day, extend that attitude to everyone you meet. Practice cherishing the simplest person like clerks or attendants or people you dislike.

Continue this practice no matter what happens or what anyone does to you.

These thoughts are simple, inspiring and helpful. The practice of cherishing can be taken very deeply if done wordlessly, allowing yourself to feel the love and appreciation that already exists in your heart.

"Seek to do brave and lovely things which are left undone by the majority of people. Give gifts of love and peace to those whom others pass by." Parmahansa Yogananda

The Saint and the Scorpion *by Swami Kripalu*

IT WAS 8:00 IN the morning. Countless pilgrims were bathing in the holy waters of the Ganges. Among them was an aged ascetic saint who had dunked himself five times, reciting each time, "Ganga Hara. Praise to Lord Shiva and the Holy River Ganges."

Before the saint had finished bathing, however, he saw a scorpion drowning in the river. His tender heart was filled with compassion.

"That poor scorpion," he thought. "It's going to die."

He knew the scorpion was poisonous and would definitely sting him if he touched it. But being a true lover of religion, he fearlessly approached the scorpion, lifted it into his cupped hands, and swiftly and skillfully threw it toward the riverbank.

The scorpion immediately stung him.

The saint's hand burst into flames, but he ignored the excruciating pain. The scorpion fell short of the riverbank, though, because the sting had taken strength from the saint's hand.

Quickly the saint approached the scorpion again. This time there were pilgrims watching from the riverbank.

"Reverend saint! " They called. "What are you doing? Let it die! What's the purpose of saving it?"

The saint said nothing.

He took the scorpion into his cupped hands a second time and threw it toward the riverbank. The scorpion stung him again. The painful flames, already blazing in his hands, were made worse by the second sting. Yet the saint ignored the discomfort again: he was an ascetic, an embodiment of tolerance itself. Sighs slipped from the mouths of the people on the bank.

"Reverend saint!" They cried again. "Why are you making this useless effort? Even though the scorpion is almost dead, it hasn't given up its instinct to sting!"

Once again, the saint said nothing.

The scorpion was still not on shore, so the saint waded a third time over to the scorpion, scooped it up into his cupped hands and threw it toward the shore.

The scorpion delivered a third ungrateful sting. But at last, the saint's efforts were successful. His eyes flooded with joy and his lips formed a sweet smile. Then he turned to the pilgrims on the riverbank and said,

"If this poisonous creature hasn't renounced its instinct to sting, even at the threat of death, why should I, a saint, renounce my instinct to serve living beings?"

"Grandfather, Great Spirit, fill us with light. Teach us to walk the soft earth as relatives to all that lives." A Lakota Prayer, Native American

Delight In Waking Up *by Yogi Amrit Desai*

Believe in the goodness of your soul.
Acknowledge how well it has guided you.
And yet know that you will fall asleep along the way.
When you sleep,
Take no delight in blaming yourself.
Take delight in waking yourself up once more.
Self-blame is the deepest injury,
The deepest sleep of all.
Wake yourself up with gentle affection.

"If your compassion does not include yourself, it is incomplete."
Jack Kornfield

66

I Am Spirit *by Deepak Chopra*

ALTHOUGH MY PHYSICAL EXISTENCE is confined to space and time, my awareness is not limited to that. I am aware of the whole field as a play of creation and destruction. Matter and energy come and go, flickering in and out of existence like fireflies, yet all events are held together and made orderly by the deep intelligence that runs through all things.

I am one aspect of that intelligence. I am the field unfolding itself in local events. My spirit is experiencing the material world through the lens of perception, but even if I see and hear nothing, I am still myself, an eternal presence of awareness.

In practical terms, this realization becomes real when no outside event can shake your sense of self. A person who knows himself as spirit never loses sight of the experiencer in the midst of experience. His inner truth says, "I carry the consciousness of immortality in the midst of mortality."

"The witnessing soul is like the sky. The birds fly in the sky but they don't leave any footprints. The one who is awakened lives in such a way that he leaves no footprints...he never looks ahead; he ever looks back; he lives in the moment." OSHO

The Dream Keeper *by John Mundahl*

*S*OMEWHERE INSIDE YOUR HEART *your dream lies waiting. If you're not sure how to find your dream, ask the Dream Keeper. Her heart is the sun. Her eyes are the stars. Her voice is the wind. And she will whisper your dream into your ear.*

Once, long ago, there was a little girl who could talk to the birds. When she was little, she was happy. She walked in the forest and played by the stream and never thought about her purpose in life. But as she grew older, she asked: Why am I here? Where am I going? Who am I?

But no one could answer these questions, so one day she walked into the forest. Maybe the birds will know, she thought. They are my friends and I will talk to them. Look at how they live. There is no hesitation in their flight. There is no hesitation in their song. Surely they know their purpose. Maybe they know mine, too.

She walked until she saw a beautiful eagle.

"Eagle," she asked. "What is your purpose?"

"To fly above the earth," the eagle replied. "From there I can see all things. Here is my feather. Fly with me."

Next she saw a hawk.

"Hawk," she asked. "What is your purpose?"

"To be a messenger," the hawk replied. "I bring news of things to come. Here is my feather. Listen to my call."

Then a tiny hummingbird flew by.

"Hummingbird," she asked. "What is your purpose?"

"To love the flowers," the hummingbird replied. "My wings are their music. Here is my feather. Hold it close to your heart."

Then she saw a graceful swan.

"Swan," she asked. "What is your purpose?"

"To live in beauty," the swan replied. "Though the water is muddy, I see only my reflection. Here is my feather. Live in peace."

The girl sat down next to a river. The sunlight warmed the water and it was beautiful, but she was sad.

"I know the purpose of all the birds," she said, "but what is my purpose?"

Then a dragonfly with wings like paper flew by. The dragonfly saw the girl was sad and wanted to help her.

"And you, dragonfly," the girl finally asked. "What is your purpose?"

"To help people find their dreams," the dragonfly replied.

"Help me, then," the girl said. "I wish to know my dream."

"You must visit the Dream Keeper," the dragonfly said. "She will tell you. She lives nearby."

The girl looked around. There was no path anywhere. There was no one calling her name. The only noise was the sound of the river going over the rocks.

"Where is her house?" The girl asked.

"The wind will tell you," the dragonfly replied. "Listen to the wind." Then the dragonfly few away.

The girl stood up. She listened for the wind, but the air was still. Then a soft breeze blew in the trees and she followed the breeze into the forest. Finally the breeze stopped and the forest was still.

"Dream Keeper?" The girl asked softly. But there was only silence. Then the grass quivered and the leaves rustled and a voice as beautiful as spring whispered, "Ask your question."

"I know the purpose of all the birds," the girl said, "but what is my purpose?"

"To find your dream and follow it," the Dream Keeper replied.

"Then tell me my dream," the girl said. "You're the Dream Keeper."

"Come closer and I will whisper your dream into your ear. But you must be still. Listen. Listen. Hush."

The girl felt the breeze blow gently, gently, Oh, so gently into her waiting ear, and with a smile she recognized now and forever the voice of the Dream Keeper. Then, from within her own heart, she heard the music of the hummingbird and she saw the beauty of the swan in the water and she heard the sharp call of the hawk and she flew with the eagle high above the earth and she knew her dream and she followed it and she was happy.

"What each must seek in his life never was on land or sea. It is something out of his own unique potentiality for experience, something that never has been and never could have been experienced by anyone else." Joseph Campbell

68

Yoga, A Gift From The Sages
by Swami Rajarshi Muni

IN INDIA FROM TIME IMMEMORIAL, many great sages devoted their entire lives to studying the secrets of human nature and existence. They pursued this search with iron endurance. They completely withdrew themselves from the commotions of the world and concentrated all their efforts solely upon this pursuit

Ultimately, their dedicated efforts bore fruit. They discovered the deepest secrets of life and the mysteries of being. They discovered a hidden most path leading upward to freedom and emancipation. Collectively they named it yoga.

Yoga is neither a religion by itself nor part of any other religious system. Yet it is around the practice of yoga that the great religions of the world developed. Great persons in these religions…call them saints, mystics, yogis, Sufis… obtained glimpses of spiritual experiences through arduous training and discipline that basically resembles yoga. They then expressed, in their own words, that the soul is immortal and emerges from some source higher and greater than itself.

"I bow with reverence to the many forms of the eternal God, the source of all beauty. I don't condemn any name or image of God. They are all worthy of worship. All the religions of the world lead to the holy feet of God, so to disrespect any religion, saint or scripture is a great insult to Him." Swami Kripalu

From Nothing To Everything Just As It Is

by Nancy Ann James

I'LL NEVER FORGET the first time I sat for Zen meditation in a suburban basement. With about one minute
of instruction in the meditation posture, and considerable
qualms about being able to sit still for one 40-minute period, let alone the standard two, I found myself breathing slowly in the prescribed cross-legged position and
thinking,

"Now what?"

I berated myself for talking to myself, but couldn't
stop. Every time I thought thoughts, as if to tell someone
later, I silently yelled at myself,

"Who cares?" I knew that all my life I had been carrying on a lively internal monologue that absolutely no one
was interested in and now was the time to shut up. So I
told myself,

"Shut up! So what? Who cares?" Over and over.

Suddenly, tears formed and began to slide down my
cheeks. I realized that this was the first time in my whole
life that I had stopped *to just plain be with myself,* the first
time I had given myself permission to simply be. I had
spent my life running and doing and trying to live up to
other people's expectations and suddenly here I was, alone
with myself, just sitting, just being, no expectations, listening to nothing at all.

The two 40-minute periods, separated by a 10-minute
slow walk, passed faster than I had dreamed possible. Instead of experiencing agonizing impatience, I was startled
when the bell rang announcing the end of each sitting period. I was sorry it ended. As soon as I could get out of

the room, I hurried to the bathroom, closed the door, and sat sobbing for about ten minutes.

I had never been so in touch with myself. I was full of pity and feeling for this poor person who had never stopped long enough to feel her body or her breath, to know her true self. I was hooked on Zen.

"It doesn't happen all at once…you become. It takes a long time."
Margery Williams

A Prayer For The Powerless

by Sister Mary Ann Kelley

Let us join our hands and hearts together and raise our voices as one in a Prayer for the Powerless:

We pray for our sisters in Africa and elsewhere who are being raped and brutalized by war.

We pray for our children here and abroad who are being born with AIDS with no chance for a meaningful life.

We pray for our elderly, those who held us and cared for us when we were young, and who now lie lost and confused from Alzheimer's and other illnesses.

We pray for our animal friends, our little brothers and sisters, who are being raised on factory farms and used in medical experiments in the name of science.

We pray for all life forms that have lost their homes in the rain forests of the world.

We pray for all living things in our air, seas, lakes and rivers that have lost their lives to human contact.

We pray for all members of our world family who have been marginalized by prejudice of any kind and thus have been denied a full life.

We, who have been given so much, join our hands and hearts together and raise our voices as one to tell those who are suffering that they are not alone, and to ask those in power, or those who seek power, to use it not for personal gain, but for the good of all life on earth.

Peace. Peace. May there be Peace everywhere.

What Is The Root? *by Hafiz*

What
Is the
Root of all these
Words?

One thing: love.

But a love so deep and sweet
It needed to express itself
With scents, sounds, colors
That never before
Existed.

"Thousands of candles can be lit from a single candle, and the life of the candle will not be shortened. Happiness never decreases by being shared." The Buddha

Consciousness *Is* Love *by Dr. David Frawley*

THE BASIC URGE of consciousness is to unite. It consists of our efforts and energies to unite either outwardly with the world or inwardly with our true nature. To be is to be related through consciousness.

Through consciousness we relate to the world and the world relates to us, not merely superficially but at a heart level. Through love's capacity for sympathy and rapport, consciousness creates devotion and compassion, the guiding powers of the spiritual life.

Consciousness is the basis of love, which is the essential attitude and energy of the heart. In fact, consciousness *is* love. On individual consciousness the Divine Consciousness projects its power of eternal and unbounded love. Love derives from consciousness, which is its home.

Consciousness is the love at the core of our being. In its internal fount of love, we find complete and perfect happiness, which arises through being able to be one with the object of our love.

"Love is patient and kind. It is not jealous or conceited or proud. Love is not ill mannered. It does not seek its own advantage and is not irritable. Love does not keep a record of wrong, is not happy with evil, but rejoices in the truth. Love is always ready to excuse, to trust, to hope, and to endure." St. Paul

Lord, Cast Your Sweet Gaze On Me

by Swami Kripalu

ONCE A SAINT CAME to a town in India.
"My brothers and sister," he said. "Anger is a demon. Don't be angry with each other. When this demon enters your mind, it creates pain and suffering in others. Give up your anger."

A certain man was in the audience and he was moved by this discourse.

"I'll give up anger!" He said to himself with great conviction. *"I will do this!"*

He walked up to the saint afterwards and said,

"Your message went deep into my heart. I won't be angry anymore!"

The saint wasn't impressed. He knew such a vow was impossible and yet he didn't want to discourage the man, either. So he gently raised his hand and blessed the man.

"Yes, but do it gradually," the saint said. "Little by little, let go of your anger."

"What do you mean?" The man said. "Why should I do it slowly? I'll just push it out and be rid of it!"

"Yes, do that, then," the saint said, remaining calm. "Just push it out and be rid of it."

"I will!" the man said. *"I'm finished with anger!"*

The man left and went home.

When he got home his wife had left a bowl of milk in the middle of the floor and the man stepped on it by mistake and spilled it. Immediately he got angry.

"Where are you?" He shouted to his wife.

His wife came running into the room and saw the spilled milk.

"Why did you leave this milk here?" The man demanded.

"I was getting some milk and the baby fell out of the crib," she said. "She cried, so I left the milk right there and ran to take care of the baby."

Now the man felt ashamed.

"I just promised that saint I wouldn't be angry anymore and here I am angry already. And over nothing, too."

So he repeated his vow all over again, with even greater conviction:

"Anger is a demon! I won't be angry anymore!"

Then he thought,

"Now, how can I remember that? I know. I'll make a sign."

So he made a sign for himself with big letters that said:

One Should Not Be Angry. Anger Is A Demon.

He wrote the words on a board and put the board on his desk at work. Now he was happy.

But later that day he started arguing with someone at work and he got so angry he hit the man with the board.

"Sometimes only God can remove our faults. We're too weak on our own. Then we should pray to Him: 'My Lord, You're the destroyer of all the demons. Let Your grace fall upon me. Hold my hand and take me to Your lotus feet.'" Swami Kripalu

74

ChooseYin *by Sister Mary Ann Kelley*

O UR PLANET WILL BE SAVED by women, not men. Men think they can solve their problems through violence. Jesus, Gandhi, and other great souls knew that men have no fear of violence—they've been killing since Cain and Abel. So they conquered men by acting like women. They brought yin to the planet, not more yang, and that's how our planet will be saved.

You can do this, too. Choose yin. Start small. *Decide to harm no living thing, including yourself, in thought, word or deed for one hour.* Then extend it for two hours. Then perhaps for an entire morning.

You'll have every reason not to do this. We live in an aggressive, angry world and our first impulse is to strike back. Jesus could have summoned Heavenly Beings in a massive show of force, totally justified, to kill those who were about to kill him, but he didn't. Gandhi blessed the man who shot him. That was their greatness. They chose yin, not yang, in a world that mocks gentleness.

"I can choose peace, rather than this." From *A Course In Miracles*

Whenever You Watch the Mind *by Eckhart Tolle*

WHENEVER YOU WATCH the mind you with-draw consciousness from the mind forms, and it then becomes what we call the Watcher, or the Witness Consciousness.

Consequently, the Watcher—Pure Consciousness beyond form, becomes stronger and the mental formations become weaker. When we talk about watching the mind we are personalizing an event that is truly of cosmic significance: Through you, consciousness is awakening out of its dream of identification with form and withdrawing from form. This foreshadows, but is already a part of, an event that is probably still in the distant future as far as chronological time is concerned. This event is called the end of the world.

"Yoga is the negation of the thought-composed mind. Then the seer abides in his own nature." The Yoga Sutras of Patanjali

The Perfect One *from the Bhagavad-Gita*

"Like the ocean,
Day by day receiving floods from all the lands,
Yet never overflows,
Its boundary line not leaping and not leaving,
Fed by the rivers but unswelled by those.
So is the Perfect One!
To his soul's ocean
The world of sense pours streams of witchery.
They leave him as they find him,
Without commotion,
Taking their tribute,
But remaining sea."

In Celebration Of Morning Light

by John Mundahl

Come, my love,
The morning light
Has found the mountain meadow.
The sleepy grass
Yawns and stretches
Nudged by love
And kissed by rosy lips.
Who would not want
To awaken to such a love?
A love like this
Is sweet and kind,
Soft and never rushed.
Each morning
It whispers
With fresh breath
To the silent grass:
    "Wake Up!
    Wake Up!
    From joy you came.
    In joy you live.
    To joy you shall return again."

"A bird does not sing because it has an answer. It sings because it has a song." A Chinese Proverb

A Christian Prayer for Peace

The Prayer of St. Francis of Assisi

Lord, make me an instrument of your peace.
Where there is hatred…let me sow love.
Where there is injury…pardon.
Where there is doubt…faith.
Where there is despair…hope.
Where there is darkness…light.

Where there is sadness…joy.

Divine Master,
Grant that I may not so much seek
To be consoled…as to console
To be understood…as to understand.
To be loved…as to love.
For it is in giving that we receive.
It is in pardoning that we are pardoned.
It is in dying that we are born to eternal life.

A Hindu Prayer for Peace *author unknown*

Oh God,
Lead us from the unreal to the Real,
Lead us from darkness to light.
Lead us from death to immortality.
Peace, Peace, Peace to all.
May there be peace in celestial regions.
May there be peace on Earth.
May the waters be appeasing.
May herbs be wholesome.
May trees bring peace to all.
May all beneficent beings bring peace to us.
May all things be a source of peace to us.
And may Thy peace itself, bestow peace on all
And may that peace come to me, also.

80

A Zoroastrain Prayer for Peace *author unknown*

We pray to God to eradicate all the misery in the world:
…that understanding may triumph over ignorance.
…that generosity may triumph over indifference.
…that trust may triumph over contempt.
…and that truth may triumph over falsehood.

81

A Baha'i Prayer for Peace *author unknown*

Be generous in prosperity and thankful in adversity.
Be fair in judgment and guarded in thy speech.
Be a lamp unto those who walk in darkness,
And a home to the stranger.
Be eyes to the blind,
And a guiding light unto the feet of the erring.
Be a breath of life to the body of humankind,
A dew to the soil of the human heart,
And a fruit upon the tree of humility.

A Buddhist Prayer for Peace *author unknown*

May all beings everywhere plagued
With sufferings of body and mind
Quickly be freed from their illnesses.
May those frightened cease to be afraid,
And may those bound be free.
May the powerless find power,
And may people think of befriending one another.
May those who find themselves in a fearful wilderness:
    The children,
    The aged,
    The unprotected,
Be guarded by beneficial celestial Beings,
And may they swiftly attain Buddhahood.

A Jain Prayer for Peace *author unknown*

Peace and Universal Love are the essence
Of the Gospel preached by all Enlightened Ones.
The Lord has preached that peace is the dharma.
I forgive all and let all creatures forgive me.
I extend love to all and hatred to none.
Know that violence is the root cause
Of all the miseries in the world.
Violence, in fact, is the knot of bondage.
"Do not injure any living being."
This is the eternal and unalterable way of spiritual life.
A weapon, however powerful,
Can always be superseded by a superior one,
But no weapon can, however,
Be stronger than love.

A Muslim Prayer for Peace *author unknown*

In the name of Allah, the beneficent, the merciful:
Praise be to the Lord of the universe
Who has created us
And made us into tribes and nations
That we may know each other,
Not that we may despise each other.
If the enemy inclines towards peace,
Do thou also incline towards peace,
And trust God,
For the Lord is the one who
Heareth and knoweth all things.
And of the servants of God,
Most gracious are those who walk on the earth in
humility,
And when we address them, we say,
"Peace."

A Native American Prayer for Peace

author unknown

Grandfather, Great Spirit, all over the world
The faces of living ones are alike.
With tenderness they have come up
Out of the ground.

Look upon your children that they may
Face the winds and walk the good road to
The Day of Quiet.

Grandfather Great Spirit,
Fill us with the Light.
Give us the strength to understand,
And the eyes to see.
Teach us to walk the soft Earth as relatives
To all that live.

The Corner Of Hollywood And Vine

by John Mundahl

I met a saint once, downtown L.A.,
In a small auditorium where she was giving a talk.
I don't remember what she said,
Just her eyes as I gave her a flower.
They came from a place foreign to me,
Great peace amid a noisy world.

She took my flower and smiled,
And I knew for one moment
That I was everything to her,
That I was all she saw,
And a tiny candle
Long buried
And forgotten
Deep within
My frozen
Heart,

Lit.

And I knew that I had worth
Just the way I was.

Later that night, when I left the auditorium,
I hugged the first beggar I saw
On the corner of Hollywood and Vine
And I went home happy.
I can still see his confused face.

"The purpose of life is to increase the warm heart. Think of other people. Serve other people sincerely. No cheating." The Dalai Lama

A Beautiful Continuation *by Thich Nhat Hanh*

WHEN WE LOOK at an orange tree we see that season after season it spends its life producing beautiful green leaves, fragrant blossoms, and sweet oranges. These are the best things an orange tree can create and offer to the world. Human beings also make offerings to the world every moment of our daily lives, in the form of our thoughts, our speech and our actions. We may want to offer the world the best kinds of thought, speech and action that we can—because they are our continuation, whether we want it to be so or not. We can use our time wisely, generate the energies of love, compassion and understanding, say beautiful things, inspire, forgive, and act to protect and help the Earth and each other. In this way, we can ensure a beautiful continuation

"Hatred does not cease by hatred, only by love. This is the eternal rule." The Buddha

The Buddha's Discourse on Good Will

May all beings be filled with joy and peace.
May all beings everywhere,
    …the strong and the weak,
    …the great and the small,
    …the powerless and the powerful,
    …the short and the tall,
    …the subtle and the gross,
    …the seen and the unseen,
    …dwelling far off or nearby,
    …being or waiting to become,
May all be filled with lasting joy.

Let no one deceive another. Let no one anywhere despise another,
Let no one out of anger or resentment wish suffering on anyone at all.
Just as a mother with her own life, protects her child, her only child, from harm,
So within yourself let grow a boundless love for all creatures.

Let your love flow outward through the universe,
To its height, its depth, its broad extent,
A limitless love, without hatred or enmity.

Then as you stand or walk, sit or lie down,
As long as you are awake,
Strive for this with a one-pointed mind;
Your life will bring heaven to earth.

"Hatred ever kills, love never dies…such is the vast difference between the two. What is obtained by love is retained for all time. What is obtained by hatred proves a burden for it increases hatred." Gandhi

I Will Leave Yoga Class Rested And Still

by John Mundahl

I will leave yoga class rested and still,
In touch with my breath,
My heart open,
Thankful I'm alive.
Breathing in,
I am a mountain, a rock, a tree,
Firmly grounded in my inner Essence.
Breathing out,
I am a flower, gentle, sweet and tender.
I wish no harm on any living thing.

My gift to the world
Is a peaceful heart,
And I give it now,
In this moment,
All that ever is
And all that ever will be.

"The heart's the essence, words only the accident." Rumi

The Sky Hunter *by Hafiz*

Keep ringing the bell,
Playing the tamboura, calling for Him.
For you have touched something holy inside
With your spirit-body,
And now your eyes look broken
Without His sacred presence near.

The heart is like that: blessed and ruined
Once it has known Divine beauty.

Then it becomes a restless sky hunter.
The lover keeps circling in their being,
Their sweetest moments with God,
Needing to kiss his face again.

"Yoga has brought peace into my life. I always know when it's time to sign up for another class." Anonymous

Brother Sun, Sister Moon *by St. Francis of Assisi*

Be praised, my Lord, with all Your creatures,
Especially Brother Sun,
By whom You bring us the day and who brings us the
light.
Fair is he and shines with a very great splendor…

Be praised, my Lord, for Sister Moon and the stars,
Which You have set clear and lovely in heaven.
Be praised, my Lord, for Brother Wind,
And for air and cloud, calms and all weather…

Be praised, my Lord, for Sister Water,
Who is very useful and humble and precious and clean.
Be praised, my Lord, for Brother Fire,
Through whom You give us light in darkness,
And he is bright and pleasant and very mighty and
strong.

Be praised, my Lord, for our Sister Mother Earth,
Who sustains us and keeps us,
And brings forth fruits and flowers of many colors and
leaves.
Praise and bless the Lord and thank Him,
And serve Him with great humility.

*"Keep close to nature's heart…and break clear away once in awhile
and climb a mountain or spend a week in the woods. Wash your
spirit clean."* John Muir

Humility Is Perpetual Quietness Of Heart
  by T.T. Carter

Humility is perpetual quietness of heart.
It is to have no trouble.
It is never to be fretted or vexed.
Or irritated, or sore, or disappointed.

It is to expect nothing,
To wonder at nothing that is done to me,

To feel nothing done against me.

It is to be at rest when nobody praises me,
And when I am blamed and despised.

It is to have a blessed home in myself,
Where I can go in and shut the door,
And kneel to my Father in secret,
And be at peace, as in a deep sea of calmness,

When all around me and above me is troubled.

"When one experiences truth, the madness of finding fault with others disappears." Goethe

A Meditation On Healing Another

by John Mundahl

SIT QUIETLY. Close your eyes. Take a few deep breaths. Picture someone you know who needs healing. Maybe it's a friend. Maybe it's a family member. Maybe it's someone at work. Their pain may be physical, emotional, or psychological.

See their face clearly. What color is their hair? What are they wearing? Are they smiling? Are they sad? Are they stressed?

Now picture a beam of light coming out of your forehead. Let it travel through the air, like a laser beam, and connect to the forehead of the person you are helping. Intensify the beam. Make it stronger. See the light shimmering and glistening, shining like the sun. Now allow the beam to descend into their chest and explode like a star all through their body filling them with healing energy.

When you are ready, open your eyes.

Enlightenment *by Eckhart Tolle*

THE WORD ENLIGHTENMENT conjures up the idea of some super-human accomplishment, and the ego likes to keep it that way. But it is simply your natural state of felt oneness with Being. It is a state of connectedness with something immeasurable and indestructible, something that almost paradoxically, is essentially you, and yet is much greater than you. It is finding your true nature beyond name and form.

The inability to feel this connectedness gives rise to the illusion of separation, from yourself and from the world around you. You then perceive yourself, either consciously or unconsciously, as an isolated fragment.

Fear arises and conflict within and without becomes the norm.

"My life has no purpose, no direction, no aim, no meaning and yet I'm happy. I can't figure it out. What am I doing right?" Charles Schultz, creator of Peanuts cartoon

Contraction and Expansion *by Swami Rama*

THERE ARE TWO LAWS in life: contraction and expansion. The contraction of your personality makes you selfish; you cannot grow. You just want to fulfill your wishes, regardless of how they affect others. Loneliness and sadness follow upon contraction. Thinking only of the little self becomes a serious problem in life.

Expansion allows your awareness to increase its knowledge of reality. You have to be prepared for expansion. Your thinking processes won't lead you to this realm; you must purify yourself so that your innermost consciousness can speak to you from its silence.

"Know ye not that the spirit of God dwelleth within you?" I *Corinthians 3:16*

96

Release The Need To Save People

by Sanaya Roman

YOU CAN DISSOLVE OBSTACLES to love by releasing the need to save people from their problems. You can love others as your soul does by allowing them to be responsible for their own lives. Taking care of others, worrying about their lives, and solving their problems can occupy so much of your attention and emotions that you have no energy left to put into your own life and spiritual path.

When you stop saving others, you can release any resentment you might feel for all the time and energy you spent on them. When you save others, you can become a victim when they do not use your help in the way you would like, when they continue to create similar problems, or when they expect and demand that you continue to save them.

Learn to recognize when you are helping others because you feel that they do not have the strength or ability to solve their own problems. When you feel an urge to help people in a way that will "save" them or take away their lessons, stop! You may find that your desire to help others really comes from your own need to feel better and to have less concern and worry about their problems.

Assume that people have the ability to solve their own problems, even if you can't see how they will. While your soul is interested in assisting people, it does not interfere with their lives. It allows people to have their own ideas, to live in whatever way they choose, to learn from their mistakes and to achieve their own successes.

"Sometimes pain and suffering are necessary. No one can grow for us." Author unknown

Wherever A Lamp Goes *by Swami Kripalu*

Wherever a lamp goes it sheds its light.
Wherever a flower goes it sheds its fragrance.
So also spread your love wherever you go.

Try to live your life like that.
Just love.
Wherever you go,
Just spread your love.
Just keep your candle of love going.
Whenever you find a candle unlit, light it up.
Get it going, everywhere.

There's no other way than that.
Remember this principle.
Hold on to this principle.
All answers lie with love.
Suffering is all that's left after losing love.

"Scatter joy." Ralph Waldo Emerson

A Meditation On Breathing *by Margaret Koblasova*

S IT QUIETLY and bring your awareness within. Close your eyes and relax the space between your eyebrows. Take a long breath in, beginning slowly. Notice the pause at the top of the breath, then let it go, long and easy, aware of the peace in the pause at the bottom of the breath. And take another breath in… and let it go.

Notice your chest rise with each inhalation and fall with each exhalation as a reassuring rhythm. In our silence, we become aware of still deeper rhythms- our heartbeat, perhaps the pulsing of the fluid in our spinal cord, the circulation of our blood, the patterns of neural communication, the actual respiration in our cells. We have the colors of our thoughts and the song in our heart. All these rhythms and melodies fold together into a beautiful symphony. This is a symphony that is uniquely yours.

Pause. Listen. Remember.

Your symphony is a part of the music of the universe. It is fully, intensely, wonderfully alive. It breathes. As you inhale, the universe is exhaling into you this vivid aliveness, this music. As you exhale, you accept it.

Resting On A Mountain Ledge *by John Mundahl*

I fell asleep today on a mountain ledge,
In Utah,
Near Moab,
Where the Colorado cuts the canyons.
My bed was Navaho sandstone.
Overhead, only blue sky, no clouds,
And nothing to break the silence except a distant crow.

Everything was still:
    The vaulted canyons.
    The ancient rocks.
    The distant mountains covered with snow.
Everything except my shattered mind
Which raced on like a bully
Determined to deny me a quiet moment.

But then,
As if in pity,
(Or perhaps from sheer indifference),
The silence of 100 million years of rock and wind and
rain
Told my mind: That's enough!
And dealt the frothing tyrant a death blow,
And I, too, lie still,
My eyes closed,
Asleep like a child.

The Great Depth is all there is.
Seek it out.
Become its friend.
Rest your head there
And fall asleep.

"I let go of what I am…I become what I might be." Lao Tse

A Precious Human Life *by the Dalai Lama*

Every day, think as you wake up,
Today I am fortunate to have woken up,
I am alive.
I have a precious human life.
I am not going to waste it.
I am going to use all my energies to develop myself,
To expand my heart out to others,
To achieve enlightenment for the benefit of all beings,
I am going to have kind thoughts towards others,
I am not going to get angry,
Or think badly about others,
I am going to benefit others as much as I can.

"If the only prayer you say in your whole life is 'thank you,' that would suffice." Meister Eckhart

A Wise Being Lives Inside Of You *by Shakti Gawain*

THERE IS A WISE BEING that lives inside of you. It is your intuitive self. Focus your awareness into a deep place in your body, a place where your "gut feelings" reside. You can communicate with it by silently talking to it, making requests, or asking questions. Then relax, don't think too hard with your mind, and be open to receiving answers. They are usually simple and relate to the present moment, not the past or future, and they feel right.

Though the messages of the intuitive self may come through a bit at a time, if we learn to follow the supply of information piece by piece, the necessary course of action will unfold. As we learn to rely on this guidance, life takes on a flowing, effortless quality. Our life, feelings, and actions interweave harmoniously with those of others around us.

Trust the deepest feelings that you get and act on them. If they are truly from your intuition, you will find that they lead to a feeling of greater aliveness and power and more opportunities begin to open up. If you don't feel more alive and empowered, you may not have been truly acting from your intuition, but from some ego voice in you. The ego seeks what it knows, the familiar, the unchangeable. Often it is based on fear. On the other hand, your intuition never comes from feelings of fear. Go back and ask for clarification and trust your intuition to give you direction.

We strive so hard to make our lives the way we want them to be. As you begin this day, imagine that you can give up struggling for a whole day. Relax for a while, and trust that your needs will be met by the natural flow of life. The philosophy of being here now and letting go of attachment is a freeing experience. When you do this, you discover that you're really perfectly okay. In fact, you feel quite wonderful. You can just let yourself be, let the world be, and give up the struggle of trying to change things.

"I call intuition cosmic fishing. You feel the nibble and then you have to hook the fish." R. Buckminster Fuller

Our True Heritage *by Thich Nhat Hanh*

The cosmos is filled with precious gems.
I want to offer a handful of them to you this morning.
Each moment you are alive is a gem,
Shining through and containing Earth and sky,
Water and clouds.

It needs you to breathe gently
For the miracles to be displayed.
Suddenly you hear the birds singing,
The pines chanting,
See the flowers blooming,
The blue sky,
The white clouds,
The smile and the marvelous look
Of your beloved.

You, the richest person on Earth,
Who have been going around begging,
Stop being the destitute child.
Come back and claim your heritage.
Enjoy your happiness
And offer it to everyone.
Cherish this very moment.
Let go of the stream of distress
And embrace life fully in your arms

"Keep your face to the sunshine and you cannot see the shadows.
It's what the sunflowers do." Anonymous

The Fawn *by John Mundahl*

Once I pulled my canoe up along a river bank
To rest a bit and stretch my legs from morning paddle.
Spring, it was, and lilac scent filled the quiet woods.
I walked toward nearby log to sit and have my morning
meal, but as I did,
I almost stepped upon a spotted fawn.

The little one lie curled, hiding in the grass,
completely still.
I moved away, thinking she might bolt and hurt herself.
She was trembling, I could see that, and dared not look
at me,
So I kept my distance.

But then the thought that I had caused her fear
To tremble so like that caused me to tremble, too,
in sudden grief.
The thought struck hard and would not leave my frozen
throat.
So I paused, and looked back, more for me than her,
Hoping for I know not what.

"Little one," I choked, "I wish you well, no harm."
I could think of nothing more to say and barely that.
But she must have heard,
Because she turned her tiny head
And looked at me with large dark eyes
And her trembling stopped,
And so did mine.

*"Let us walk softly on the Earth, with all living beings great and
small, remembering as we go that one God, kind and wise, created
all." A Cherokee Blessing, Native American*

Keepers *author unknown*

I GREW UP in the '50s with practical parents. A mother, God love her, who washed aluminum foil after she cooked in it, then reused it. She was the original recycle queen, before they had a name for it.

My father was happier getting old shoes fixed than buying new ones. Their marriage was good, their dreams focused. Their best friends lived close by. I can see my parents now...Dad in trousers, tee shirt and a hat...and Mom in a house dress, lawn mower in one hand, dishtowel in the other.

It was the time for fixing things. A curtain rod, the kitchen radio, screen door, the oven door, the hem in a dress. We kept things. It was a way of life and sometimes it made me crazy. All that re-fixing, eating, renewing. I wanted just once to be wasteful. Waste meant affluence. Throwing things away meant you knew there would always be more.

But then my mother died, and on that clear summer night, in the warmth of the hospital room, I was struck with the pain of learning that sometimes there isn't any more. Sometimes what we care about most gets all used up and goes away...never to return.

So while we have it...it's best to love it...and care for it...and fix it when it's broken...and heal it when it's sick.

This is true for marriage and old cars and children with bad report cards, and dogs with bad hips and aging parents and grandparents. We keep them because they're worth it, because we're worth it.

"You can search the whole universe and not find a single being more worthy of love than yourself. Since each and every person is so precious to themselves, let the self-respecting harm no other being." The Buddha

The Saint Who Couldn't Practice What He Preached

by Swami Kripalu

O NCE THERE WAS a rich man in India with only one son. The rich man grew old and one day his son died. The old man cried so heavily that he couldn't stop. Relatives and friends came to his side and tried to console him, but nothing worked. He just kept crying and crying. Soon his friends started thinking that if we can't get him to stop crying, he'll die soon, too.

There was a great learned man living in the town, a saint, well respected by everyone. His words and presence were powerful so several relatives of the old man went to the saint and asked for his help.

"Please help us," they said. "Our dear relative is so distraught over the death of his son that he won't stop crying. Perhaps you could explain to him the nature of death and help him overcome his loss."

"Yes, I can do that," the saint said. He was very confident. "I'll visit him and everything will be alright."

When the saint approached the house of the rich man, he could hear the old man crying loudly inside. The saint knocked on the door. The rich man knew about the visit and opened the door, quieting down for a moment. He gave the saint a seat and then burst into tears again, wailing loudly in front of the saint.

"This death has occurred by the will of God," the saint said sweetly. "You must accept it. The soul of your son is eternal, undying. He lives still in soul form. This body is like a garment of clothes. Just as we change clothes, so we change our form at death, that's all. Your son is still alive and you will see him again."

The saint kept talking like this, very sweetly, explaining all the beautiful things from the Shastras and other scriptures. The businessman finally quieted down and stopped crying.

Two years went by. The businessman got over the death of his son and became busy with other activities in his old age. Then one day he happened to pass by the house of the saint again. There was a large crowd of people outside the door.

"What's going on here?" The old man asked. "What's wrong? Why are you all standing here looking so worried?"

Before anyone could answer, however, the old man heard someone crying loudly inside. He recognized the voice of the saint and realized the saint was crying uncontrollably about something. He was stunned. How could someone as learned and wise as this saint be crying so loudly over anything?

So he went inside and found the saint wailing loudly in deep pain and sorrow.

"Dear sir?" He asked softly. "Why are you crying like this?"

"I've been suffering from tuberculosis now for two years," the saint replied. "A kind doctor advised me to drink goat's milk to help my condition, so I bought a goat and drank her milk each day. It was such a wonderful goat and today she died."

"You're crying over a dead goat!" The old man asked incredulously.

"Old man," the saint said. "The wife who died was yours, but the goat was mine!"

"Without laughter, there would be no Tao." Lao Tze

A Meditation On Cosmic Justice *by John Mundahl*

S IT QUIETLY. CLOSE YOUR EYES. Take a few deep breaths. Picture someone who has hurt you. Remember the incident clearly. Where were you? What happened?

Now remind yourself that whatever this person did to you, will happen to them. This is cosmic law. Whatever we sow, we will reap. We cannot escape the consequences of our actions. You do not have to be involved with this anymore. Let it go. Give it up to cosmic justice. You do not have to like this person. You do not have to forget what happened to you. Just release the thought to strike back. All will be settled with perfect justice in due time by a higher power.

When you are ready, open your eyes.

The True Peace *by Black Elk, Native American*

The first peace, which is the most important
Is that which comes within the souls of people
When they realize their relationship,
Their oneness, with the universe and all its powers
And when they realize that at the center
Of the universe dwells the Great Spirit
And that this center is really everywhere,
It is within each of us.
This is the real peace,
And the others are but reflections of this.
The second peace is that which is made between two individuals,
And the third is that which is made between two nations.
But above all, you should understand that there can never
Be peace between nations until there is known that true peace,
Which, as I have often said, is within the souls of men.

"An eye for an eye makes the whole world blind." Gandhi

Last Respects *author unknown*

ONE DAY THE EMPLOYEES of a large company returned from their lunch break and were greeted with a sign on the front door. The sign said: "Yesterday the person who has been hindering your growth in this company passed away. We invite you to join the funeral in the room that has been prepared in the gym."

At first everyone was sad to hear that one of his or her colleagues had died, but after a while they started getting curious about who this person might be. The excitement grew as employees arrived at the gym to pay their last respects. Everyone wondered:

"Who is this person who has hindered my progress? Well, at least he or she is no longer here!"

One by one the employees got closer to the coffin and when they looked inside they became speechless. They stood over the coffin in shocked silence as if someone had touched the deepest part of their soul.

There was a mirror inside the coffin. Everyone who looked inside the coffin could see himself or herself. There was also a sign next to the mirror that said: "There is only one person who is capable of limiting your growth; it's YOU."

You are the only person who can revolutionize your life. You are the only person who can influence your happiness, your realization and your success. You are the only person who can help yourself.

Your life doesn't change when your boss changes, when your friends change, when your parents change, when your partner changes, when your company changes. Your life changes when you change, when you go beyond your limiting beliefs, when you realize that you are the only one responsible for your life.

The most important relationship you can have is the one with yourself.

The Angel Of Struggle *by Swami Kripalu*

Today you have all gathered to celebrate my birthday. It's the start of my 67th year and I bless you with all my heart. I'm an old seeker wanting only final liberation.

You call me Dada, or Grandfather, and it isn't proper for me to cry in front of you, but every word I speak, every gaze from my eyes, is full of love for you. I don't speak English, but can any language truly express love? No, love is expressed only through the heart and the eyes.

Life is the flow of our own existence between birth and death. Some people say this is an endless circle of mistakes, which can never be prevented, or that life is a chaotic mixture of happiness and unhappiness.

Other people take a different view. They say that life means love; life means progress; life means light; life means evolution.

Both groups agree, however, that life means struggle, that we all must struggle.

This world is a battlefield. Anyone born has to be a warrior, whether you're a boy or girl, man or woman, young or old, king or beggar, literate or illiterate, saint or sinner, our major dharma or duty in this world is to fight.

The compassionate Lord has one special Angel to help with our fight. This is the Angel of Struggle. Just as our food won't digest properly without exercise, so too our life won't develop properly without struggle. The outward form of struggle may appear cruel, but its inner nature is not malicious. She enters our life without invitation and does whatever she pleases, but she blesses us with true knowledge, the knowledge we each need at that time in our life.

How skillful she is! What a beautiful sculptor!

"If you can find a path with no obstacles, it probably doesn't lead anywhere." Frank A. Clark

Our Notion Of Death *by Thich Nhat Hanh*

A DROP OF RAIN falling on the ground disappears in no time at all. But it is still there somehow. Even if it is absorbed into the soil, it's still there in another form. If it evaporates, it's still there in the air. It's become vapor; you don't see the drop of rain, but that doesn't mean it's no longer there. A cloud can never die. A cloud can become rain or snow or ice, but a cloud cannot become nothing. To die means from something we become nothing, from being we pass into nonbeing. That is our idea of death. But meditation helps us to touch our true nature of no-birth and no-death. Before the cloud manifests as a cloud, the cloud has been water vapor, has been the ocean. So it has not come from nonbeing into being. Our notion of birth is just a notion. Our notion of death is just a notion.

That insight is very important; it removes fear. When we understand that we cannot be annihilated, we are liberated from fear. It is an immense relief. With non-fear, true happiness is possible and so is peace. And if you are at peace, our civilization may also find peace.

"The end of birth is death. The end of death is birth. This is ordained." The Bhagavad-Gita

Mother and Child *by Yogi Amrit Desai*

See a child inside mother's womb.
Child has nothing to do.
Mother provides all.
Child breathes mother's breath.
Child feeds from mother's food.

You are in the womb of the cosmic Mother,
Divine Shakti.
Live in ultimate oneness with her.
Receive all her gifts.
Mother does it all for you.

You do not even have to grow.
Mother takes care of all.
Trust that everything you strive for will be taken care of,
In the absence of your fighting, your worrying.
Feel the warmth of the Mother.
Feel the warmth of her Love.

"Intense love does not measure. It just gives." Mother Teresa

Put Your Inner Female In The Guiding Position

by Shakti Gawain

E ACH OF US, man or woman, has within us an inner male and an inner female. The inner female acts as your intuition, the door to your higher intelligence. Your male listens to her and acts to support her feelings. The true function of male energy is to provide absolute clarity, directness and a passionate strength based on what the universe inside of you, coming through your female, tells you.

In order to live a harmonious and creative life, you need to have both your inner female and male energies fully developed and functioning correctly together. To fully integrate the inner male and female, you need to put your female, your intuition in the guiding position.

The female power, the power of the spirit, is always within us. It is up to the male energy, the ego, to determine how we relate to that power. We can fight it, block it, attempt to control it, try to keep ourselves separate from it, or we can trust and open up to it, learn to support it and move with it. Individually and collectively, we are shifting from a position of fear and control to a position of surrender and trust of the intuitive.

We may not realize that the basic functions of feminine and masculine energies exist in each person. We usually associate male and female energies with their respective body types. From this perspective each person would be only half a person, dependent on the other half for its very existence. As we cannot live effectively in the world without the full range of masculine and feminine energies, each sex has felt helplessly independent on the other for its survival. Now, as we are becoming aware of both male and female qualities within us, a deep sense of wholeness can emerge for each individual.

Traditionally, men have been disconnected from their female energy, thereby disconnected from life, power and love. Men have been out there in the world secretly feeling helpless, alone and empty, although they must pretend to be in control and powerful. They seek nurturing and inner connection through women, but as they connect with their own inner female, they receive her incredible love from within themselves.

Traditionally, women have been in touch with their female energy—intuition and feelings—but they haven't backed her up with their male energy. Many have not acknowledged what they know inside. They have acted as if they were powerless when they are really powerful. They have sought external support and validation from men. As women claim their inner male and allow him to support their female energy, they feel both feminine and powerful.

"Know the masculine. Keep to the feminine." Lao Tzu

Don't Let It Die An Orphan *by John Mundahl*

Follow others
Until you're tired of their exhaust,
Then strike out on your own.
Become friends with your playful self again,
That part of you
The world snatched away
When you weren't looking.
Choose a different future,
Not the one that looms
As some grim sentence,
But the one that nags to you
In quiet moments.
Don't let it die an orphan.

"Is the system going to flatten you out and deny you your humanity, or are you going to use the system to the attainment of human purposes?" Joseph Campbell

Your Journey Inward *by Swami Rama*

Only through meditation
Can the human personality fully unfold,
For then one meets his or her real self.
It is a journey without movement.
Along the way
You cast aside
All the opinions and appraisals
With which others have labeled you.
Behavior is the effect of thought,
And thought stimulates emotion.
Your journey inward
Must travel past everything
That moves in the thought realm.
Meditation means
You are becoming independent of this world.

"When you find the truth, you will not change the universe. Only you change. You begin with you. You travel with you. You arrive with you. The journey to truth is from the alone to the alone."
Yogi Amrit Desai

The Good News *by Thich Nhat Hanh*

The good news they do not print.
The good news we do print.
We have a special edition every moment,
And we need you to read it.
The good news is that you are alive,
That the Linden tree is still there,
Standing firm in the harsh winter.
The good news is that you have wonderful eyes
To touch the blue sky.
The good news is that your child is there before you,
And your arms are available: hugging is possible.
They only print what is wrong.
Look at each of our special editions.
We always offer the things that are not wrong.
We want you to benefit from them and help protect
them.
The dandelion is there by the sidewalk,
Smiling its wondrous smile,
Singing the song of eternity.
Listen. You have ears that can hear it.
Bow your head. Listen to it.
Leave behind the world of sorrow, of preoccupation, and
get free.
The latest good news is that you can do it.

"I believe in life after birth." Maxie Dunham

Shy One *by John Mundahl*

In the still hours of the morning,
When I sit with you, I know you love me,
And tenderness towards all swells and bursts
Within my heart like a tulip bud in spring.

But then the day takes you away
And I walk alone again in busy world.
I hide my wound with smiling face and wonder
If and when we'll meet again.

I know you haven't left me.
I know it's I who have left you.
Yet the world pounds my mind and body
With heavy hand and drives you from my heart

Shy One,
Hold me close.
Keep your tender eyes upon me.
Remember me, your child, when the world tears us apart.

"God regards with merciful eyes not what you are, or what you've been, but what you wish to be." Author unknown

Oh, Great Spirit, Whose Voice I Hear In The Winds

translated by Chief Yellow Lark

Oh, Great Spirit
Whose voice I hear in the winds
And whose breath gives life to all the world,
Hear me. I am small and weak.
I need your strength and wisdom.
Let me walk in beauty and make my eyes ever behold
The red and purple sunset.
Make my hands respect the things you have
Made and my ears sharp to hear your voice.
Make me wise so that I may understand the things
You have taught my people.
Let me learn the lessons you have
Hidden in every leaf and rock.
I seek strength, not to be greater than my brother,
But to fight my greatest enemy, myself.
Make me always ready to come to you
With clean hands and straight eyes,
So when life fades, as the fading sunset,
My Spirit may come to you without shame.

"Take only memories. Leave nothing but footprints." Chief
Seattle, Native American

Wooden Bowls *author unknown*

A FRAIL OLD MAN lived with his son, his daughter-in-law and his four-year-old grandson. His eyes were blurry. His hands trembled and his step faltered. The family ate together nightly at the dinner table, but the elderly grandfather's shaky hands and failing sight made eating difficult. Peas rolled off his spoon dropping to the floor. When he grasped his glass of milk, it often spilled clumsily at the tablecloth.

With this happening almost every night, the son and daughter-in-law became irritated with the mess.

"We must do something about grandfather," the son said.

The daughter-in-law agreed. "I've had enough of his milk spilling, noisy eating and food on the floor," she said.

So the couple set up a small table in the corner of the kitchen. Grandfather sat alone there while the rest of the family enjoyed their dinner at the main table. Since grandfather had broken a dish or two, his food was served in wooden bowls. Sometimes when the family glanced in grandfather's direction, he had a tear in his eye as he ate alone. Still, the only words the couple had for him were sharp scoldings when he dropped a fork or spilled food.

The four-year-old watched all this in silence.

One evening before supper, the father noticed his son playing with wood scraps on the floor.

"What are you making?" He asked the child sweetly.

"Oh, I'm making a little wooden bowl for you and mama to eat your food from when I grow up," the child answered innocently and went back to work.

The parents were speechless. Then tears streamed down their cheeks. Though no words were spoken, both knew what must be done. That evening the husband took grandfather's hand and gently led him back to the family table.

For the remainder of his days grandfather ate every meal with the family and neither husband nor wife cared any longer when a fork was dropped, milk was spilled, or the tablecloth was soiled.

"The worst prison is a closed heart." Pope John Paul II

Practicing Silence *by Deepak Chopra*

PRACTICING SILENCE MEANS making a commitment to take a certain amount of time to simply Be. Experiencing silence means periodically withdrawing from the activity of speech. It also means periodically withdrawing from such activities as watching television, listening to the radio, or reading a book. If you never give yourself the opportunity to experience silence, this creates turbulence in your internal dialogue.

Set aside a little time every once in a while to experience silence. Or simply make a commitment to maintain silence for a certain period each day. You could do it for two hours, or if that seems a lot, do it for a one-hour period. And every once in a while experience silence for an extended period of time, such as a full day, or two days, or even a whole week.

What happens when you go into this experience of silence? Initially your internal dialogue becomes even more turbulent. You feel an intense need to say things. I've known people who go absolutely crazy the first day or two when they commit themselves to an extended period of silence. A sense of urgency and anxiety suddenly comes over them. But as they stay with the experience, their internal dialogue begins to quieten and soon the silence becomes profound. This is because after a while the mind gives up. It realizes there is no point in going around and around if you—the Self, the spirit, the choice-maker—are not going to speak, Period. Then, as the internal dialogue quietens, you begin to experience the stillness of the field of pure potentiality.

"Everything worthwhile for the soul is gained through silence. When you verbalize, you've moved into your head." Yogi Amrit Desai

---

120

You May Have Heard That God Is In Us
by Thich Nhat Hanh

YOU MAY HAVE HEARD that God is in us, or that the Buddha is in us. But for most of us this is an abstract notion. We have such a vague idea of what Buddha or God actually is. In the Buddhist tradition, Buddha resides inside us as energy—the energy of mindfulness, the energy of concentration and the energy of insight. This is what brings about understanding, compassion, love, joy, togetherness and nondiscrimination.

Some of our friends in the Christian tradition speak of the Holy Ghost, or the Holy Spirit, as the energy of God. Wherever the Holy Spirit is, there is healing and love. We can speak in the same way of mindfulness, concentration and insight. The energy of mindfulness, concentration and insight gives rise to understanding, compassion, forgiveness, joy, transformation and healing. This is the energy of the Buddha.

If you are inhabited by that energy, you are a Buddha, at least for that moment, and that energy can be cultivated and can manifest fully in you.

"Undisturbed calmness of mind is attained by cultivating friendliness toward the happy, compassion toward the unhappy, delight in the virtuous, and indifference towards the wicked." The Yoga Sutras of Patanjali

Sick With Fever *by John Mundahl*

Today I'm sick with fever.
Yes, I know,
We struck a deal on that morning,
Long ago, in early dawn,
That you would sweep my house,
Sweep it clean,
And leave not a speck of dust remaining,
And I would yield.
I remember.
I haven't forgotten.
But today I'm sick with fever.

Yes, I know,
You wish to plug each hole
In the colander of my soul
So that I can hold your wine,
But each hole dies hard,
An old friend who hastens not to leave,
And today I'm sick with fever.

Yes, I know,
Each cut you take from ego flesh
Is with a tender knife,
But still it hurts,
And today I'm sick with fever.
Let me rest.
Let me rest.

"This yoga, I say, cometh not lightly to the ungoverned ones. But he, who by master of himself, shall win it, if he stoutly strives thereto." The Bhagavad-Gita

The Disciple Who Almost Drowned

by Swami Kripalu

T HERE ONCE WAS A man who was looking for a guru. He was a serious devotee, but he had not found a guru to his liking yet. He had visited many saints in India, but he had always left unsatisfied.

His question to each saint was the same.

"How can I create a burning desire for God, one that will bring immediate results?"

No saint he visited could answer this question to his satisfaction.

One day, by chance, Ramakrishna Paramahansa, the Guru of Swami Vivekenanda was near by. This devotee asked around and found Ramakrishna. He was walking next to a river.

"Kind, sir," the devotee asked sincerely, "How can I create a burning desire for God, one that will bring immediate results?"

"Son," Ramakrishna replied sweetly. "I can't give you that answer here on the bank of the river. But come with me into the water and I can give it to you there."

"I will do that," the devotee replied. "I'll go with you."

Ramakrishna took the man's hand and gently led him into the river. Deeper and deeper they went. Then suddenly with great force, Ramakrishna pushed the man's head under the water and held it there and wouldn't let him up! The man struggled and kicked and drank water trying to breath. Finally, just before the man drowned, Ramakrishna grabbed the man by his hair and pulled him up.

"Save me! Save me!" The man screamed. "I'm drowning!"

"That's a burning desire," Ramakrishna said sweetly. "We have to cry to God from deep pain, then God will save us."

"Yoga is possible for anybody who really wants it. Yoga is universal…but don't approach yoga with a business mind looking for worldly gain." Sri Krishna Pattabhi Jois

It Is Peace *by Barb Larson Taylor*

What does stillness sound like?
What does it sound like when you
Turn off the television set and cell phone?
What does it sound like when you
Take a break from talking
With family, friends and colleagues?
What does it sound like in your mind when you
Turn off the constant stream of thoughts?
What does stillness sound like?

What does stillness feel like?
Does it feel uncomfortable?
Unfamiliar?
Rejuvenating?
Calming?
What does stillness feel like?

What would happen if you stopped thinking about the
past?
Stopped replaying the same tapes over and over in your
mind?
What would happen if you stopped thinking about the
future?
Always waiting with anticipation for what is next?
What would happen if you brought your focus to this
moment?
This breath coming in…
This breath going out…

What is this?
When you hear stillness,

When you feel stillness,
When your focus is only on this moment?

It is Peace.

"By nature we are travelers toward perfection. What is perfection? To become what you already are! Death is simply a habit of the body, not of your essence." Swami Rama

Offer Your Heart *by Yogi Amrit Desai*

As you love yourself,
Love comes through you.
Offer that love to everyone you meet today.
Bring yourself closer to someone.
Bring someone closer to you.
As you offer yourself to someone,
You offer your heart to yourself.
Love is not an isolated incident
Practiced with a certain person
During a certain time of day.
Love is using every opportunity
To bring someone closer to your heart.
Treat each person
As if God has come to teach you
Through that person.
As you learn to be fully present
And accepting of each person you meet,
You transform yourself.
You learn to embrace
And love the whole universe

"A single rose can be my garden...a single friend, my world." Leo
Buscaglia

125

All Life Is Yoga *by Dr. David Frawley*

ALL LIFE IS YOGA, which means unification. We are all striving according to our understanding to become one with the real, the good, and the source of happiness. All individual life aims consciously or unconsciously at re-integration with the Cosmic Life. We are all striving to expand our frontiers and increase our connections in order to find wholeness and peace. Yoga is not a new path to follow but a way to become conscious of the original impetus of life. Yoga is the movement and evolution of Life itself.

All psychological problems arise ultimately from a misapplication of the energy of consciousness. Instead of uniting with the eternal inner reality in which is lasting joy, we attach ourselves to transient external objects whose fluctuations bring pain. The practice of Yoga, or inner integration, reverses all psychological problems by merging the mind back into its immutable source of pure consciousness, in which resides perfect peace.

"Yoga is integrative. Ego is separative. Separation is at the core of all human suffering. Integration-yoga-is the ultimate solution."
Yogi Amrit Desai

Choose Your Part, Then *by John Mundahl*

When the lights in the theatre go down,
And the curtain goes up
And the play begins,
It cannot be stopped by me.
Only the Director can do that.
But I can choose my part.
What will it be?

A comedy?
A tragedy?
A mystery?
A fantasy?
A pleasure cruise?
A competition?
A search for truth?
A boring experience?
A jail?
An adventure?
A playground?
A chance to change?
A search for love?
A bank account?

I get to choose,
But I must choose,
Or the play will play me.
Choose your part, then,
Don't wait.
There's no sick leave
And there's no rewind.

"The play's the thing." Shakespeare

Growing Good Corn *author unknown*

THERE ONCE WAS A farmer who grew award-winning corn. Each year he entered his corn in the state fair where it won a blue ribbon. One year a newspaper reporter interviewed him and learned something interesting about how he grew it. The reporter discovered that the farmer shared his seed corn with his neighbors.

"How can you afford to share your best seed corn with your neighbors when they are entering corn in competition with yours each year?" The reporter asked.

"You don't understand how corn grows," the farmer replied. "The wind picks up pollen from the ripening corn and swirls it from field to field. If my neighbors grow inferior corn, cross-pollination will steadily degrade the quality of my corn. If I want to grow good corn, I must help my neighbors grow good corn."

This man is not only a good farmer, but he also understands the connectedness of life. His corn cannot improve unless his neighbor's corn also improves.

So it is with our lives. Those who choose to live in peace should help their neighbors to live in peace. Those who choose to live well should help others to live well, for the value of a life is measured by the lives it touches. Those who choose to be happy should help others find happiness, for the welfare of each is bound up with the welfare of all.

"I can live for two months on a good compliment." Mark Twain

Consciousness: The World Within by

Dr. David Frawley

CONSCIOUSNESS IS THE MOST wonderful thing in the universe. There is no limit to its depth or to its grasp. It is like a vast ocean, but unless we know how to navigate properly through it, we can get lost. If we dive into it without the right preparation, we can drown. Many mentally disturbed people are so immersed in their internal consciousness that they can no longer function in the external world. To us they appear caught in delusion; in fact, they may be accessing deeper realities, although not in a wholesome manner.

Consciousness is our inner world. When the yogi looks within he sees his consciousness pulsating with cosmic forces; when we look within, however, we see only darkness or vague memories. Our external vision blinds us. We are so conditioned to the vivid light of the senses that we cannot perceive the subtle light of consciousness.

Learning to observe the contents of our consciousness is the most important part of mental and spiritual development. Yoga provides specific disciplines and meditation techniques for this purpose. When consciousness is illumined, we transcend all external limitations. We no longer need to experience the external world, because we have learned its lesson—that all is within.

"Ninety-nine percent of who you are is invisible and untouchable."
R. Buckminster Fuller

The Straw On The River Ganges

by Swami Kripalu

ONE DAY THE RIVER Ganges was flowing beautifully out of the high Himalayas. The sun was bright on the pure, clean water. There was a sudden gust of wind and the wind picked up a straw and dropped it on the current of the river.

"Look at me!" The straw said. "This river is so beautiful! I'm passing flowers and woods and I can see all the mountains and overhead the sky is blue!"

The river kept flowing and passed one holy place after another.

"Look at me!" The straw said. "I'm passing all the holy places of India."

They came to a place where a lady was gathering water by the side of the river. She had a bucket and she dipped her bucket into the river and the straw went into her bucket.

"Look at me!" The straw said. "This lady will carry me throughout the town. I've found the holy place meant for me."

"Good by, straw," the river Ganges said. "I've taken you to all the holy places and I'm pleased that you found a place that you like. But first, though, don't you think you should thank me?"

"Thank you?" The straw said. "For what?"

"For carrying you," the river said. "You floated in my current and I brought you here."

"No!" the straw said. "Didn't you see my swimming? I wasn't floating; I was swimming."

"Little straw," the river laughed. "You were floating, not swimming. You did nothing on your own. You didn't have the strength to swim on your own in my water and if you had, you would have swam all over the place and not arrived at this holy spot. Go now if you want to, live here and be happy, but give thanks to God."

And the river left.

"Man, who lives in darkness, thinks 'Look at me! Look at all the things I'm doing!' Yet God is so great that He hides behind His creation. We should give thanks to Him and remember from whom we draw our strength." Swami Kripalu

A Sanskrit Salutation To The Dawn *author unknown*

Look to this day for it is life, the very life of life.
In its brief course lie all the verities and realities
Of our existence.
The bliss of growth, the splendor of beauty,
For yesterday is but a dream
And tomorrow is only a vision,
But today well-spent makes every yesterday
A dream of happiness
And every tomorrow a vision of hope.
Look well therefore to this day.
Such is the salutation to the dawn.

"I practice yoga now with gentleness, especially in the morning
before the children awake, when I can have a few moments alone
with the sunrise. That's all I need, so great is my gratitude."
Anonymous

Interdependence *by the Dalai Lama*

Right from the moment of our birth,
We are under the care and kindness of our parents,
And then later on in our life when
We are oppressed by sickness and become old,
We are again dependent on the kindness of others,
And since at the beginning and end of our lives,
We are so dependent on the kindness of others,
How can it be in the middle that
We would neglect the kindness towards others?

"It is preoccupation with possessions, more than anything else, that prevents us from living freely and nobly." Bertrand Russell

Mullah Nasrin and the Dandelions

a Sufi story, author unknown

ONE DAY A MAN named Mullah Nasrin decided to take up gardening. He loved flowers and vegetables and he became an adept gardener. But when his garden became plagued with dandelions, Mullah became more and more upset.

Finally, he couldn't take it anymore. He traveled to the palace of the king and consulted the king's own personal gardener. The royal gardener gave Mullah instructions on how to get rid of the dandelions.

Mullah returned home full of enthusiasm and followed the instructions perfectly. But still the dandelions returned.

Really angry now, Mullah returned to the king's palace and found the royal gardener.

"You're a fraud!" He hollered. "Your remedy was no better than the rest! What else can I do about these dandelions?"

The royal gardener looked thoughtful and stroked his chin. Finally he said softly,

"Mullah Nasrin, there's only one thing to do. You must learn to love dandelions."

"One day I just quit. No more workshops on self-improvement. No more things to fix in myself. I was done with it. I am what I am, I told myself, and that's the end of it and I burst into laughter and felt just fine." Anonymous

The Trip Home *by John Mundahl*

I'm calling to tell you that I'm coming home.
Yes. I'm on my way.

I have a good map; the one you gave me.
But I can't go the speed limit

All the time. It's too fast for me.
So I stopped to rest, on the Interstate,

At a rest stop, out of the heat.
The highway I'm on is hot

And today I'm your sunburned moth
Who needs to take a tanning day.

*"Let everything be allowed to do what it naturally does, so that its
nature will be satisfied." Chuang Tzu*

That Man Alone Is Wise *from the Bhagavad-Gita*

"That man alone is wise who keeps the mastery of
himself.
If one ponders on objects of the sense, there springs
attraction.
From attraction grows desire,
Desire flames to fierce passion,
Passion breeds recklessness,
Then the memory, all betrayed,
Lets noble purpose go and saps the mind,
Till purpose, mind and man are all undone.

But if one deals with objects of sense,
Not loving and not hating,
Making them serve his free soul,
Which rests serenely lord,
Lo! Such a man comes to tranquility,
And out of that tranquility shall rise
The end and healing of all earthly pains."

The Compulsive Thinker *by Eckhart Tolle*

T HE COMPULSIVE THINKER, which means almost everyone, lives in a state of apparent separateness, in an insanely complex world of continuous problems and conflict, a world that reflects the ever-increasing fragmentation of the mind.

Enlightenment is a state of wholeness, of being "at one" and therefore at peace, at one with life in its manifested aspect, the world, as well as with your deepest self and life unmanifested—at one with Being.

Enlightenment is not only the end of suffering and of continuous conflict within and without, but also the end of the dreadful enslavement to incessant thinking.

What an incredible liberation this is!

"All that happens in the mind appears to be happening to you. When you don't mind your mind, nothing is happening." Yogi Amrit Desai

The Wise Woman And The Precious Stone

author unknown

ONCE A WISE WOMAN was traveling in the mountains and found a precious stone in a stream. The next day she met another traveler who was hungry and the wise woman opened her bag to share her food. The hungry traveler saw the precious stone and asked the woman to give it to him. She did so without hesitation.

The traveler left rejoicing in his good fortune. He knew the stone was worth enough to give him security for a lifetime. But a few days later, he came back to return the stone to the wise woman.

"I've been thinking," he said. "I know how valuable this stone is, but I give it back to you with the hope that you will give me something even more precious. Give me what you have within you that enabled you to give me this stone."

Sometimes it's not the wealth we have, but what's inside us that others need.

The Broken Glass Jar *by John Mundahl*

One day my 7-year-old daughter
Came home from school in tears.
Someone had called her fat.
The wound went deep.
I called the Principal and complained.
I called the parents and complained.
Some things require a response.
Sometimes we must say:

"Stop! You can't say things like that!
You can't act that way!
You're hurting someone else!"

Nothing helped.
My daughter cried herself to sleep that night,
And so did I.
The next morning she refused to go to school,
And I refused to let her go.
I took the day off and we went to a funny movie,
Her choice,
And had popcorn,
And then we went to the park and played together
Until the hurt was gone.

Be kind to each other.
Speak gently.
Don't hurt anyone.

Once the glass jar falls from the table
It's hard to put it back together again.

"My religion is simple. My religion is kindness." The Dalai Lama

I Am There For You *by Thich Nhat Hanh*

THE MOST PRECIOUS GIFT we can give offer others is our presence. When our mindfulness embraces those we love, they will bloom like flowers. If you love someone but rarely make yourself available to him or her, that is not true love. When your beloved is suffering, you need to recognize his or her suffering, anxiety and worries, and just by doing that, you already offer some relief. Mindfulness relieves suffering because it is filled with understanding and compassion. When you are really there, showing your loving-kindness and understanding, the energy of the Holy Spirit is in you.

"I am only one, but still I am one. I cannot do everything, but still I can do something. I will not refuse to do the something I can do." Helen Keller

How Hafiz Became A Sufi *a traditional Sufi story.*

IT IS SAID when he was twenty-one and working as a baker's assistant, Hafiz delivered some bread to a mansion and happened to catch a fleeting glimpse of a beautiful girl on the terrace. That one glimpse captured his heart and he fell madly in love with her, though she didn't even notice him. She was from a wealthy noble family and he was a poor baker's assistant. She was beautiful; he was short and physically unattractive—the situation was hopeless.

As months went by, Hafiz made up poems and love songs celebrating her beauty and his longing for her. People heard him singing his poems and began to repeat them. The poems were so touching that they became popular all over Shiraz.

Hafiz was oblivious of his new fame as a poet. He thought only of his beloved. Desperate to win her, he undertook an arduous spiritual discipline that required him to keep a vigil at the tomb of a certain saint all night long for forty nights. It was said that anyone who could accomplish this near-impossible austerity would be granted his heart's desire.

Every day Hafiz went to work at the bakery. Every night he went to the saint's tomb and willed himself to stay awake for love of this girl. His love was so strong that he succeeded in completing this vigil.

At daybreak on the fortieth day, the archangel Gabriel appeared before Hafiz and told him to ask for whatever he wished. Hafiz had never seen such a glorious, radiant being as Gabriel. He found himself thinking,

"If God's messenger is so beautiful, how much more beautiful must God be!"

Gazing on the unimaginable splendor of God's angel, Hafiz forgot all about the girl, his wish, everything. He said,

"I want God!"

Gabriel then directed Hafiz to a spiritual teacher who lived in Shiraz. The angel told Hafiz to serve this teacher in every way and his wish would be fulfilled. Hafiz hurried to meet his teacher and they began their work together that very day.

"It's only when we realize that life is taking us nowhere that it begins to have meaning." P.D. Ouspensky

So Far Today *author unknown*

Dear Lord,

So far today I've done all right.
I haven't gossiped,
Haven't lost my temper,
Haven't been greedy, grumpy, nasty, selfish, or over
indulgent.
I'm very thankful for that.
But in a few minutes, God, I'm going to get out of bed,
And from then on, I'm going to need a lot more help.

"Life is either a daring adventure or nothing at all." Helen Keller

A Meditation On The Deathless Self

by Dr. David Frawley

ONE OF THE BEST meditations is to meditate upon death. This is not something morbid; it is simply facing the ultimate reality of our lives. It is very healing to all our psychological problems that revolve around our transient personal problems.

Sit or lie down comfortably. Imagine that your body is dying. Withdraw your attention from your body, senses and mind and place it in your heart. Imagine that you are a small flame in the heart of this great city of the body. Offer all your thoughts and feelings into that immortal flame. Realize that flame as the True Self, the I-Am-That-I-Am. Let everything else go. Bathe, purify and transform yourself in that pure light of awareness. See all the universe, all time and space, within it.

"Never the spirit was born. The spirit shall cease to be never.
Never was time it was not. End and beginning are dreams!
Birthless and deathless and changeless remaineth the spirit forever.
Death hath not touched it at all, dead though the house of it
seems!" The Bhagavad-Gita

Somebody Else *by Shoshannah Brombacher*

RABBI DOVID OF LELOV was walking down the street when all of a sudden a woman jumped on him and began to beat him and scream at him. After a while, she noticed that the rabbi was not the man she thought he was…her husband…who had left her to her fate and abandoned her many years ago. She burst into tears out of shame and remorse.

Rabbi Dovid got back to his feet and consoled her, saying that she had not beaten him, but she had beaten her eloped husband.

Doesn't this happen to us all the time? We get angry…at a stranger, at a friend, at a loved one…only to discover that we were never truly angry at them, but at the person we thought they were.

"We rarely experience reality. Instead we experience our reactions, which are adopted, acquired, distorted and cultivated." Yogi Amrit Desai

A Special Meal *author unknown*

ONCE THERE WAS A poor devoted woman who always prayed to the Glory of God asking little, if anything, for herself. But one thought, one desire, continued to surface in her mind, so finally she petitioned the Lord with this thought that, if it were possible, she would love to prepare a special meal and have God at her table. And God, in His love for this goodly woman, said he would indeed come the next day and share a meal with her.

Filled with ecstasy, the woman went out the following morning with her meager purse and purchased the delicacies she felt would please the Lord. Returning home, she prepared a banquet and waited patiently for her honored guest. Soon there was a knock on her door and when she opened it, there stood an old beggar asking for something to eat.

Being a woman of God, she couldn't turn the beggar away, so she invited him for something to eat. The beggar felt as if he was in a dream, such was the feast before him. He finished all the food, thanked the lady and left.

The woman was only slightly disheartened. She gathered up her purse, her coat, and hurried back to town to get more food for her special guest. Her funds were less now and so the food was not quite so elaborate. Nevertheless, she lovingly prepared another meal and awaited the arrival of God.

A few hours went by and there was a loud knock on her door. This time it was a woman beggar with no teeth, deaf, who spoke quite loudly and was rather rude, insisting that any true believer in the Lord would not deny her something to eat. Though the woman had no more money to buy more supplies, she invited the beggar woman in and offered her a seat at the table. The woman ate everything, didn't even thank her host and left without closing the door.

By now it was getting dark both inside and out. The woman's faith was strong, so even though somewhat distraught, she didn't give up, but looked around her humble house to see if there was anything she could sell in order to buy more food for God.

She hurried to town with a little silver cup that had been in her family for several generations, but she was willing to part with it for the great honor of sharing a meal with God.

Late that night she rushed home to prepare yet a third meal. She waited and waited until once again there was a knock on the door. Holding her breath, she slowly opened the door to find yet another poor man dressed as a wandering monk in search of a meal.

Again she offered hospitality, with as much grace as she could muster in her disappointment. This man also ate all the food on the table and left after blessing the woman for her kindness. The woman was so discouraged and dismayed that she could only lightly nod in thanks.

Now it was too late to buy any more food and she had no more money, anyway. She got down on her knees, weeping heart-broken tears. She asked God what she had done wrong. Why had God not come to share at her table as He had promised?

Then God, in His divine compassion and mercy, lifted the woman off her knees, and holding her close to His heart said,

"My child, I enjoyed your hospitality so much that I came three times!"

Today I Make Peace With My Body-Home

by John Mundahl

Today I make peace with my body-home.
My weight isn't perfect, but I don't care anymore.
My nose isn't perfect, but I don't care anymore.
My ears aren't perfect, but I don't care anymore.
I'm getting older, too, but I don't care anymore.
Yesterday I overate. So what? That was yesterday.

Today is here now,
And I accept my body as it is and for what it is,
A home for my soul for a few years, that's all,
And then I'll be gone.

So today I make peace with my body-home.
I'll be happy when I wake up in the morning.
I'll smile at my body in the mirror before I go off to
work.
In the evening I'll give thanks
To my feet and legs and eyes and ears
For serving me throughout the day.

And before I fall asleep,
I'll give thanks to my heart,
For opening in tenderness,
Even briefly,
Lest I forget
That we are all suffering,
That we are all visitors on this small planet
For a short, short time
And then we will all be gone.

"I exist as I am, that is enough." Walt Whitman

Be the Buddha *by Eckhart Tolle*

All cravings are the mind seeking salvation
Or fulfillment in external things and in the future
As a substitute for the joy of Being.

As long as I am my mind,
I am those cravings,
Those needs, wants, attachments, and aversions,
And apart from them there is no "I"
Except as a mere possibility, an unfulfilled potential,
A seed that has not yet sprouted.

In that state,
Even my desire to become free or enlightened
Is just another craving for fulfillment or completion in
the future.

So don't seek to become free of desire or achieve
enlightenment.
Become present.
Be there as the observer of the mind.
Instead of quoting the Buddha, be the Buddha,
Be the "awakened one," which is what the word buddha
means.

*"To dream is to try to make the external world meet your demands.
It only works in your sleep." Yogi Amrit Desai*

The Two Women *a Buddhist parable*

ONCE A BEAUTIFUL well-dressed woman visited a house. The master of the house asked her who she was and she replied that she was the goddess of wealth. The master of the house was delighted and treated her nicely.

Soon another woman appeared who was ugly and poorly dressed. The master asked who she was and the woman replied that she was the goddess of poverty. The master was frightened and tried to get her out of the house, but the woman refused to leave.

"The goddess of wealth is my sister," she said. "We have an agreement to never live separately. If you chase me out, she goes with me."

The master was so afraid of her that he put her out and when he returned the other woman had disappeared also.

Fortune goes with misfortune; birth goes with death; bad things follow good things. Foolish people dread misfortune and strive after good fortune, but wise people ignore differences of fortune and thus are not disturbed by their coming and going.

"Praise and blame, gain and loss, pleasure and pain come and go like the wind. To be happy, rest like a giant tree in the midst of them all." The Buddha

Your Sweet Voice *by John Mundahl*

The day came
When I gave away all my things,
And simplified my life,
Thinking that surely now
I could spend more time with You.
But nothing happened.
I was here, waiting, but You were someplace else.

I took my trip to India,
And visited Your home and place of birth,
And bought my Shiva statues and OM stickers,
And walked with sandaled feet along the Ganges,
But nothing happened.
I was there, waiting, but You were someplace else.

Confused and sad,
I returned home and sat outside my door
Wondering where you were?
And then you came on tiptoes,
And whispered in my ear,
Oh, so sweetly!
Oh, so sweetly!
"Go and help your neighbor weed his garden.
I am there!"

"If I keep a green bough in my heart, the singing bird will come."
A Chinese proverb

Rest At The Feet Of The Lord *by Swami Kripalu*

Pray to the Lord daily.
Accept happiness and unhappiness as the grace of the
Lord.
The Lord keeps the sun in the sky
So everyone can have heat and light
And keeps the moon in the sky
So everyone can have coolness at night.

The Lord opens the flowers
And allows them to bloom
And then closes and dries them up.

All of these things happen by the will of the Lord
And we are His children and He loves us.
He doesn't want us to suffer or to be anxious.
So rest,
Rest at His holy feet knowing you are cared for.

"Everything that I have is yours." Luke 15:31

I Turn To Thee, Blessed Mother *by John Mundahl*

Today as I lie in savasana, my yoga class over,
I turn to Thee, Blessed Mother.
You are the sweet softness that heals my body.
You are the gentle calm that cools my heated mind.
You are the one who whispers to me:
    "Open your heart, my love, to the gentle rain,
    To the beautiful flowers, to the birds that want to
    sing to you."
When I leave this class,
Hold me close,
Lest my heart close again.
Don't forget me,
Though I may forget you in the rush of my day.
Remind me always
That you are as close as my breath,
As far away as my fearful mind.
Remember me.
Don't forget me.
I am your simple child
Lost in a confusing world.

"The eternal God is your dwelling place and underneath are the everlasting arms." Deuteronomy 33:27

Take, These, My Last Words

from The Bhagavad-Gita

"Take, these, My last words, My utmost meaning have!
Precious thou art to Me, right well-beloved.
Listen! I tell thee for thy comfort this.
Give Me thy heart! Adore Me! Serve Me!
Cling in faith and love and reverence to Me!
So shalt thou come to Me!
I promise true, for thou art sweet to Me!

And let go those—rites and writ duties!
Fly to Me alone!
Make Me thy single refuge!
I will free thy soul from all its sins!
Be of good cheer!"

Ending Blessing

May it be beautiful before me.
May it be beautiful behind me.
May it be beautiful below me.
May it be beautiful above me.
May it be beautiful all around me.
In beauty it is finished.
In beauty it is finished.
Happily I go forth.

A Navajo Chant, Native American

ACKNOWLEDGMENTS

G RATEFUL ACKNOWLEDGMENT IS MADE to the following for permission to reprint material copyrighted or controlled by them. I made a thorough effort to locate all rights holders and to clear reprint permissions. Given the vast amount of knowledge floating freely on the Internet, this was difficult, at times. If I omitted any required acknowledgments or overlooked any rights, it was unintentional. Please contact me and I will rectify the error.

Amber-Allen Publishing, Inc. for *We Are Travelers On A Cosmic Journey* and *Practicing Silence* From the book *The Seven Spiritual Laws of Success* ©1994, Deepak Chopra. Reprinted by permission of Amber-Allen Publishing, Inc. P.O Box 6657, San Rafael, CA 94903. All rights reserved. For *A New Dream* From the book *The Four Agreements* ©1997, Miguel Angel Ruiz, M.D. Reprinted by permission of Amber-Allen Publishing, Inc. P.O. Box 6657, San Rafael, CA 94903. All rights reserved.

Danna Faulds for *I Am Ready*, from *ONE SOUL: MORE POEMS FROM THE HEART OF YOGA* ©2003 by Danna Faulds, published by Peaceable Kingdom Books, 53 Penny Lane, Greenville, Virginia 24440 yogapoems@aol.com. Reprinted by permission of the author.

Daniel Ladinsky for the following selections by Hafiz: *The Sun Never Says, It Felt Love, What Is The Root?, The Sky Hunter, Now Is The Time, How Hafiz Became A Sufi, The God Who Only Knows Four Words*, From the Penguin publication *The Gift, Poems by Hafiz* © 1999 Daniel Ladinsky and used with his permission.

HJ Kramer Inc. for *Release The Need To Save People* taken from *SOUL LOVE*, ©1997 by Sanaya Roman, published by HJ Kramer Inc., P.O Box 1082, Tiburon, California 94920. Reprinted by permission of publisher.

Public Domain. The following selections are more than 100 years old and *may* be public domain. Since this does not ensure that a selection is public domain, I made every attempt to find copyright and permission information on these selections, but received no responses to my inquiries. If I have errored on any selection, please contact me and I will correct the mistake: *Earth Teach Me, Oh Great Spirit Whose Voice I Hear in the Winds, The Prayer of St. Francis, Brother Sun, Sister Moon, Humility is Perpetual Quietness of Heart, The True Peace, A Sanskrit Salutation to the Dawn, The Day I Discovered the Meaning of Love.*

Random House for *I Am Spirit*, from *AGELESS BODY, TIMELESS MIND* © 1993 by Deepak Chopra, published by Three Rivers Press, a division of Crown Publishers, Inc., used by permission of Random House, Inc.

Selections by unknown authors. I took the following selections off the Internet. All were listed as "Author Unknown." I made every attempt to find permission or copyright information on these selections but found none, nor did I get responses from any of my inquiries. If you have information regarding any of these selections, please contact me and I will gladly make the correction. *Are Your Potatoes Heavy? It's Simple, The Dancer and the Starfish, Keepers, So Far Today, Heartprints, A Special Meal, Growing Good Corn, Last Respects, The Wise Woman and the Precious Stone, Wooden Bowls, A Hindu Prayer for Peace, A Zorastrian Prayer for Peace, A Baha'i Prayer for Peace, A Buddhist Prayer for Peace, A Jain Prayer for Peace, A Muslim Prayer for Peace, A Native American Prayer for Peace.*

Selections from the Bhagavad-Gita were taken from Arnold's Edition, printed in 1977 by The Self-Realization Fellowship, 3880 San Rafael Avenue, Los Angeles, California 90065.

Selections from the Buddhist Bible were taken from *The Teaching of Buddha: The Buddhist Bible*, printed by Kenkyusha Printing Company, Tokyo, Japan. 1934, with references to: American Buddhist Academy, 331 Riverside Drive, New York 25, New York. Tri-State Buddhist Church, 1947 Lawrence